ALTERNATIVE ANSWERS TO

ASTHMA
& ALLERGIES

ALTERNATIVE ANSWERS TO
ASTHMA
& ALLERGIES

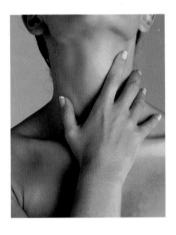

BARBARA ROWLANDS

CONSULTANT

≡People's Medical Society.

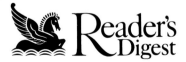

The Reader's Digest Association, Inc.
Pleasantville, New York • Montreal

A Reader's Digest Book
Conceived, edited, and designed by
Marshall Editions Ltd.
The Orangery
161 New Bond Street
London W1Y 9PA

Copyright © 1999 Marshall Editions Developments Ltd.

Library of Congress Cataloging in Publication Data

Rowlands, Barbara.
    Asthma & allergies / Barbara Rowlands ; consultant,
People's Medical Society.
    p. cm. -- (Alternative answers to)
    ISBN 0-7621-0246-2
    1. Allergy--Alternative treatment. 2. Asthma--
Alternative treatment. I. Title. II. Title: Asthma and
allergies III. Series.
    RC588.A4 R69 2000
    616.97'06-dc21
                                        99-16029

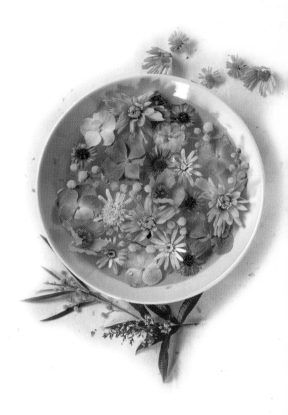

EDITORS	Richard Shaw
	John C. Miles
DESIGNER	Sue Storey
ART EDITOR	Frances de Rees
COPY EDITOR	Lindsay McTeague
MANAGING EDITOR	Anne Yelland
MANAGING ART EDITOR	Patrick Carpenter
EDITORIAL DIRECTOR	Ellen Dupont
ART DIRECTOR	Sean Keogh
PICTURE RESEARCH	Antonella Mauro
EDITORIAL COORDINATOR	Rebecca Clunes
EDITORIAL ASSISTANT	Sophie Sandy
INDEX	Laura Hicks
PRODUCTION	Nikki Ingram
DTP EDITOR	Lesley Gilbert
COVER PHOTOGRAPH	Tony Latham

Originated in Malaysia by C H Colour Scan
Printed in Italy Milanostampa Caleppio Milano

Contents

Introduction

Few of us escape allergies. Around 100 million people in the world have asthma—six percent of adults and 10 percent of children—and at least 40,000 people die from the disease each year. The world over, people are wheezing in greater numbers than ever before. Asthma is everywhere and, despite the fact that there are treatments, it's on the increase. Skin and food allergies also seem a part of modern life. Allergies to foods such as peanuts and shellfish are becoming more common, often with fatal results, and many more of us are sensitive to foods, such as milk, bread, and eggs, that were once regarded as staples.

No one really knows what is causing this epidemic, but doctors, geneticists, chemists, environmentalists, lung specialists, dietitians, and alternative practitioners now have several theories. One is that we have changed the way we live. Although it is clear that asthma and allergies run in families, there is increasing evidence that they are triggered by environmental factors. The modern centrally heated and air-conditioned home, sealed against the movement of fresh air, is the perfect environment for the house dust mite, which breeds in our carpets and soft furnishings; its droppings can trigger asthma. You may develop asthma because you were brought up in a household of smokers, or because you had a chest infection. Eczema can be triggered by stress. Some people develop allergies at work from flour, sawdust, sulfur dioxide, formaldehyde, and other industrial chemicals. You may suffer from chronic skin problems or bloating even though your diet is full of fresh fruit and vegetables. Even if you lead the healthiest of lives working in the fresh air, you can succumb to hayfever because your eyes sting and your nose streams from pollen. Some people say we're running out of fresh air, even in the more remote regions of the world. Finally we are all too clean.

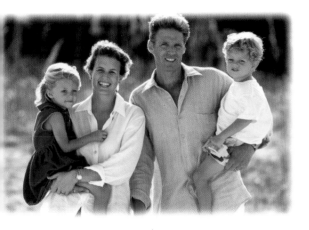

In the past our immune systems battled against a sea of dirt and in the process became strong. Now we are inoculated against common diseases and our homes are squeaky clean. With nothing much to fight against, the immune system takes up arms against the harmless house dust mite or pollen grain. Too little dirt is making us ill.

Medication can dampen down allergic symptoms and drugs can and do save lives. One injection of epinephrine can prevent death from a severe food or insect allergy. If everyone took their drugs properly there would be far fewer deaths. But many people are worried about the drugs they take and resent being so dependent on inhalers, pills, and steroid creams. Most sufferers just want to feel well.

The advice in this book is to keep taking medication but empower yourself and take responsibility for your condition. Changes in your diet, the way you furnish your home, and how you approach your work can make a difference, and there is a host of complementary therapies you can try that may improve your symptoms. Clinically controlled trials have shown that some therapies, such as homeopathy, herbal medicine, and hypnotherapy, can have direct effects on the lungs by reducing tension, relaxing tense muscles, or boosting the immune system. Such therapies are not quick fixes, the easy option when drugs fail. They require time, energy, and commitment. But used sensibly in conjunction with medication they can transform your life.

How to use this book

This book works in several ways. If you read straight through you will understand what asthma is, how complementary and conventional treatments may help asthma sufferers, and what you can do on a day-to-day basis to limit the likelihood of an attack, and cope with one. Alternatively, follow the "Find out more" references throughout the book to learn all you need to know about a specific aspect of your condition.

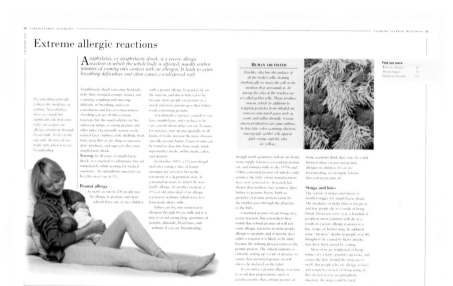

1 *Chapter One defines asthma and other allergies, explaining what they are and how they can affect the body's major systems and organs. It assesses how common they are becoming globally and pinpoints those people who are most at risk of suffering from asthma or another allergy.*

2 *Chapter Two looks at the causes of asthma and allergies and the factors that may trigger an attack or reaction. It offers practical solutions to enable you to enable you to reduce your risk of suffering – precautions include not exercising when the pollen count is high and double rinsing clothes to avoid dermatitis – and easy ways to reduce stress, a significant factor in asthma and allergies.*

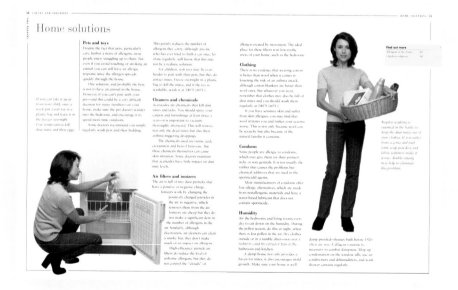

3 *Chapter Three discusses the ways in which conventional medicine has helped sufferers from asthma through drug therapy. The emphasis is on how the various drugs you might be prescribed work, and what side effects they may trigger.*

Treatments for hay fever

Many people are wary of taking drugs, particularly for something that seems as mild as hay fever. But apart from taking away the pleasure of a warm summer's day, hay fever can be debilitating, making sufferers feel tired and run down and unable to do anything without constant sneezing and coughing.

Pollen from grasses are the most common and widespread triggers of hay fever. Avoid them as much as possible during the pollen season.

Antihistamines

Antiallergy drugs

Steroids

Decongestants

Desensitization techniques

Incremental desensitization

Neutralization

Enzyme-potentiated desensitization (EPD)

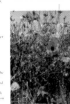

A field of wildflowers may be the source of a number of airborne allergens. It is a good idea to take your hay fever medication with you if you are going out for a walk in the country.

Find out more

Meditation

Practised regularly, meditation aims to bring about total relaxation and inner calm. Sitting quietly and breathing gently sounds simple, but in fact meditation requires an inner discipline you may initially find hard to achieve, but it is worth persevering.

Wear comfortable clothing and meditate somewhere draft free that is neither too hot nor too cold. Closing your eyes will prevent stray thoughts from disturbing your sense of inner calm.

How to meditate

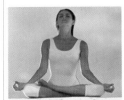

Find out more

TYPES OF MEDITATION

BUDDHIST MEDITATION	Buddhist meditation has been practiced for thousands of years. You do not use a mantra; instead you concentrate on the "mindfulness of breathing" or "awareness of in-and-out breathing" (anapana-sati), and "development of loving kindness" (metta-bhavana) toward those around you.
TRANSCENDENTAL MEDITATION	Transcendental meditation, popularized in the 1960s by the Indian yogi Maharishi Mahesh, is increasingly practiced by professionals to alleviate stress and is gaining acceptance in medical circles. There are over four million people throughout the world who use TM. During a course you will be given a mantra, or meaningless word, the silent repetition of which induces deep relaxation.
MANTRA MEDITATION	This is a meditation on a simple word or phrase. You can choose your own or it can be given to you, as in TM. It can either mean something pleasurable to you, such as "love" or "peace" or it can be meaningless. The best-known mantra is "Om," which is the most sacred word for Hindus. You should repeat the mantra regularly and silently to yourself while you meditate.
CANDLE MEDITATION	You can meditate on a lighted candle, crystal, or icon. This is a yogic form of meditation known as tratak, in which you gaze at the object for about a minute, focusing on its texture, shape, and color, then close your eyes and visualize it. Ideally, it should be at eye level and about 3 ft (1 m) away. When the image fades, open your eyes and focus on the object again.
PRAYER	Repeating prayers with the help of a rosary is another form of meditation.

---

4 *Chapter Four discusses your treatment options. While conventional medicine can keep asthma and other allergies under control, many complementary therapies have proven helpful for allergic conditions when used alongside conventional medication. These include both self- and practitioner-administered therapies.*

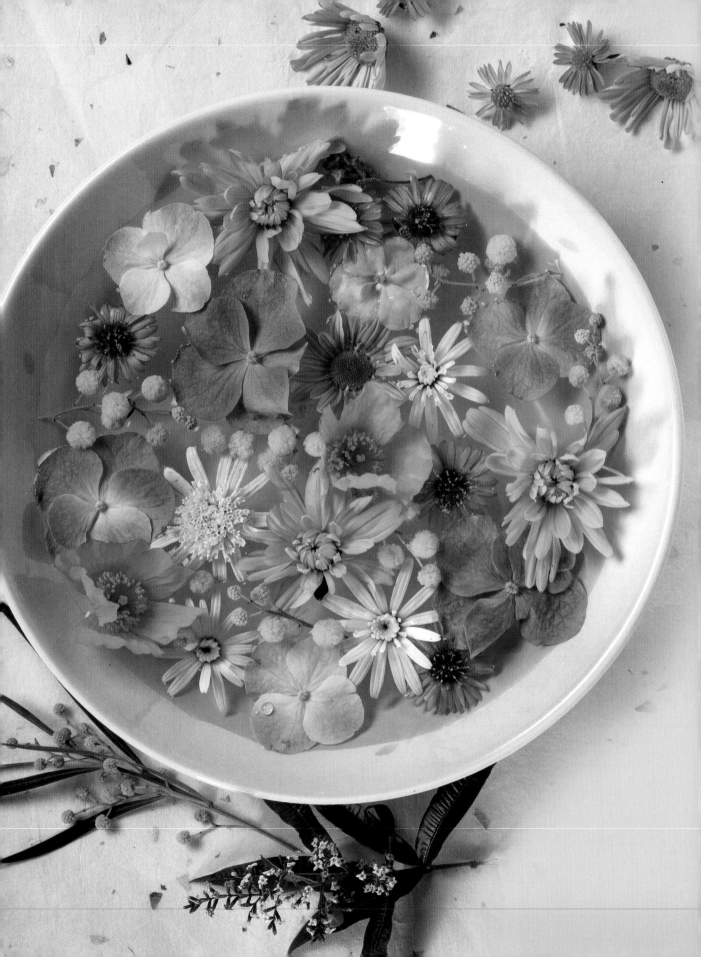

1

UNDERSTANDING

ALLERGIES

It is easy to identify an asthma attack. Its distinctive symptoms—coughing, gasping for air, and wheezing—mean that most of us would recognize an attack if we saw one. But despite this familiarity and the fact that asthma is reaching epidemic proportions, doctors cannot agree on a definition of asthma, and there is no simple test to indicate whether a person suffers from it. It is also not known what causes it, although the factors that trigger it are clear.

Asthma is just one of a number of familiar allergies, many of which are on the increase. In order to understand why so many people have miserable summers because of hay fever, or why so many children go to school with an inhaler, it is important to understand how allergies can affect the body's systems.

What are asthma and allergies?

The word "asthma" is Greek and means "to breathe hard" and that is the main symptom of asthma. If you have asthma the airways in your lungs are almost always sore and inflamed and quick to respond to anything that irritates them.

The best way to define asthma is by its four main symptoms:
• Coughing—often the first sign that an asthma attack is on the way. You may either have a dry cough or a cough with phlegm, and coughing often happens at night or after exercise.
• Shortness of breath—it is hard to finish one breath before starting another.
• Wheezing—the whistling noise made when someone having an attack breathes out. It is caused by sticky fluid—mucus—produced by the reddened and inflamed airways.
• Tightness in the chest—a feeling that you have a vice around your chest or that someone is giving you an overenthusiastic bear hug.

Triggers, such as droppings of the house dust mite and pets, can cause these airways to narrow suddenly. An asthma attack can be frightening—one sufferer described it as "a bit like drowning"—and, in extreme cases, asthma can kill.

Allergies

Allergies are very common and one in three people will have an allergy at some time during their life. One in five of us has hay fever and one in every six children has a skin condition, usually eczema.

An allergy is your body overreacting to something that is normally harmless. Most people can walk past freshly cut grass, cuddle up to the family pet, and happily munch their way through a bag of peanuts. A bee sting usually causes no more than a flash of pain and a red lump. For most people drugs, such as antibiotics or local anesthetics, cause no problems. But if you have an allergy many of these things do and the allergic reaction —like an asthma attack—can be sudden and violent.

Very rarely, allergies can kill. For a tiny number of people, if they do not get the right medication immediately, a bee sting or a peanut can mean death.

The most common allergies
• Asthma
• Hay fever and itchy eyes
• Rashes and skin conditions such as eczema and dermatitis
• Food allergy
• Wasp- or bee-sting allergy

THE AIRWAYS AND ASTHMA

In an asthma attack the airways that take air from your nose or mouth to the lungs become constricted, making it hard to breathe. The problem may be caused in three different ways: the airway walls become swollen; the muscles of the airways go into spasm; mucus collects and obstruct the airways.

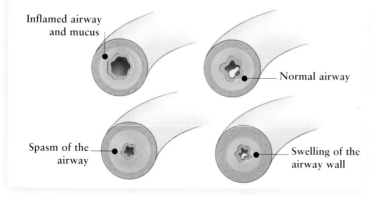

Inflamed airway and mucus

Normal airway

Spasm of the airway

Swelling of the airway wall

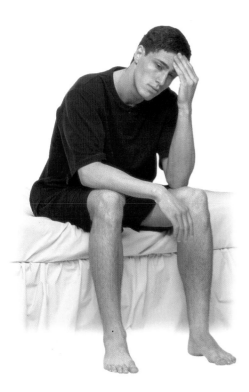

If you have nocturnal asthma you may cough without waking or wheeze periodically. Sitting up sometimes helps.

Types of asthma

There are two main types of asthma. The first is allergic asthma, sometimes called extrinsic asthma, and 9 out of 10 asthma sufferers fall into this group. This means that you—or someone in your family—is allergic to one or more common allergens.

The second type is nonallergic asthma, or intrinsic asthma, of which doctors do not really know the causes—there is no history of the disease in your family, and you do not seem to be allergic to anything. In either case your asthma may be mild, moderate or severe, and if it has been going on a long time it is "chronic."

Then there is "brittle" asthma, which is very rare. In this case you may have a sudden attack, usually brought on by an allergy, which comes out of the blue and is difficult to control. Finally, there is night-time or nocturnal asthma.

Hay fever

Every spring and summer hay fever affects tens of millions of people. At the height of the hay-fever season up to one third of us will show a positive reaction to a skin test using extracts of grass pollen.

Hay fever—or to give it its more accurate name, seasonal allergic rhinitis— is not caused by hay, nor does it cause a fever. It is an allergy to airborne pollen from trees, grass, and plants, as well as mold spores. Some people are allergic to just one or two types of pollen; others are sensitive to several. In northern Europe, grass pollen is the major cause of hay fever. Allergic rhinitis is generally characterized by sneezing and a runny or blocked nose, often accompanied by itchy, watery eyes. Sufferers may feel unattractive, grumpy, tired, run down, and unable to concentrate. It prevents many from enjoying a good meal, and the constant sniffling and sneezing take the enjoyment out of kissing. It may even put a damper on sex.

You can develop hay fever at any age, but it normally makes its appearance between 8 and 20, and rarely after 40. Men are more likely to have hay fever than women and, contrary to popular belief, it seems to be more common in cities and towns than in the countryside.

Hay fever rates have increased fourfold over the past 20 years, despite falling pollen counts associated with the reduction of grassland. Scientists say that vehicle exhaust pollution is sensitizing the airways of hay fever sufferers, making them more prone to allergies.

Proteins on the pollen grains are washed off and stick to particles in the polluted air, which, because they are so small, are breathed deeply into the lungs, increasing the risk of allergic reaction. ▶

What are asthma and allergies?

Thousands of teenage hay-fever sufferers fare worse academically than nonsuffering peers. Inability to concentrate, sore itchy eyes, and a runny nose all contribute to their poor results.

Is asthma like bronchitis?

Diagnosing asthma is notoriously difficult, particularly in children. Asthma is sometimes missed simply because its symptoms are like those of bronchitis.

Bronchitis is an inflammation of the air passages, or bronchi, and is marked by one of asthma's main symptoms – wheezy breathlessness. In acute bronchitis, the inflammation is caused by an infection, usually a virus; chronic bronchitis is caused by pollution, often tobacco smoke. People with bronchitis may wheeze and cough, but they do not have asthma.

Babies are prone to wheeziness and may sometimes be diagnosed as having asthma when in fact it is a passing chest infection. Croup, caused by a virus, may seem similar to asthma. Your baby may wheeze and cough and although it usually clears up after a week, it does recur.

Asthma in childhood

More and more children seem to be affected by asthma. There is an explosion in the number of cases of childhood asthma—in some countries the number of children with

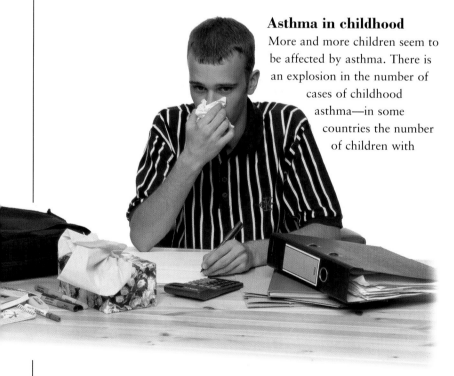

asthma has doubled in a generation. This means increased numbers of hospital admissions, lost school days, and millions of children on medication. In Western countries an average of one in seven schoolchildren has asthma and almost a third of children under five have had one attack of wheezing.

The most common triggers of asthma in childhood are exercise and infections—asthma sparked off by allergies is relatively rare. Most very young children have attacks of asthma brought on by a cold or a virus. Typical symptoms are wheezing and/or coughing, particularly at night, after colds, and after exercise. This can be frightening, even if in the majority of cases childhood asthma is mild and can be easily controlled. Nevertheless, many children do have sudden attacks that are extremely distressing.

If your child has allergic asthma, your family may have a tendency toward atopy, that is, be prone to allergies. You may not have asthma, but you may have hay fever or eczema. If you are allergy-free then you will probably find that your mother or father, your partner's parents or either set of grandparents have allergies.

Smoking and childhood asthma

In one survey of 10,000 children carried out in 1996, 7 out of 10 said smokey places made their asthma worse and a third lived with someone who smoked. Children of mothers who smoke more than 10 cigarettes a day are twice as likely to get asthma as the children of nonsmoking mothers.

Few children and teenagers die from asthma, but they account for half of all hospital admissions. The good news is that two-thirds of children grow out of their asthma.

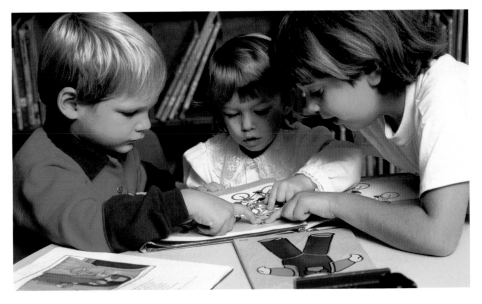

Asthma and allergies in small children have become alarmingly common. In every classroom at least one child is likely to be taking some form of medication, and in some areas as many as one in five may have asthma.

Asthma in adults

Some adults have had asthma since childhood, but usually it appears out of the blue. Some may have had a touch of it when they were children and then no sign of it for 20 or 30 years; others will never have had asthma before.

The disease may be triggered by a new allergen, such as an irritant that you have come across in a new job or a new household pet. Some drugs, such as beta-blockers and aspirin, can trigger asthma. Other triggers in adulthood include chest infections and stress. Asthma symptoms get worse in 4 out of 10 women from 7 to 10 days before menstruation.

The over-50s

Nearly half of asthma sufferers do not develop the illness until they are over 50, and most deaths from asthma happen in people over 45. Asthma may be more serious if it happens when you are older.

Late-onset asthma, as it is called, is much less likely to be triggered by allergies than by colds, the flu, viral infections, and irritants such as tobacco smoke. A snap of cold weather could set off an attack. It is more common in men than women.

Allergies in children

In general, allergies such as asthma are on the increase. One in six children has a skin condition, such as eczema, brought on by an allergy. One person in 20 suffers from raised itchy lumps called urticaria (hives) and one in five has hay fever. More people seem to have food allergies than before, and many people are being stricken with sick building syndrome.

Childhood illnesses caused by allergies include eczema, asthma, hay fever, itchy eyes, and allergic rhinitis. Children in small families, particularly the first born, have more allergies than those in large families simply because their immune system, with which the body fights off infection, is not as effective in resisting allergies. In large families, viral infections are readily passed from one child to another, and these children seem to suffer from fewer allergies.

A global overview

Around 100 million people in the world have asthma—roughly 6 percent of adults and 10 percent of children—and asthma is on the increase. At least 40,000 people die from the disease each year. Australia is at the top of the asthma league, with the United Kingdom and New Zealand coming close behind.

Asthma is more common in cities and towns than rural areas. Research shows that it is on the increase, with the greater number of newer patients being among children and young people.

This is true of most industrialized countries. A study in Australia showed that the number of children who used some form of medication for asthma rose from 7 percent in 1982 to 25 percent 10 years later. In some countries almost 30 percent of children have asthma.

Across the developed world more and more people of all ages are being admitted to the hospital with the symptoms of asthma, despite the fact that the overall standard of living has increased and people are generally healthier and living longer. It is not just happening in countries with a dense population and large towns. The figures are the same for Australia, New Zealand, the US, Scandinavia, the United Kingdom and other industrialized Western European countries.

CASE HISTORY

Fiona Paton, her husband, and their two children, 13-year-old Simon and 11-year-old Kirsty, live in a town north of London, England—asthma capital of Europe.

Simon began having asthma when he was an 18-month-old baby, but it was a manageable condition until he started school.

"There was a heavy buildup of traffic with parents dropping off their children close to school," says Fiona. "We walked to school, but by the time we got there Simon had difficulty breathing and would have to use his inhaler. At home any dust would cause him to wheeze."

Soon Simon was having attacks twice a week. He had to see a specialist every month and was a regular visitor at the local hospital. On several occasions, Fiona had to nebulize him—pump steroids into his lungs to keep his airways open.

"When you have a child with asthma there is so much to think about," says Fiona. "You have to keep everything in his bedroom dust-free, but then he'll have an attack if he walks into a dusty classroom or a friend's house. We have to consider what to wash the clothes with and how best to avoid friend's pets.

"Fortunately now that Simon is older, he is able to make decisions for himself, and knows what he can and can't do. His asthma is manageable again."

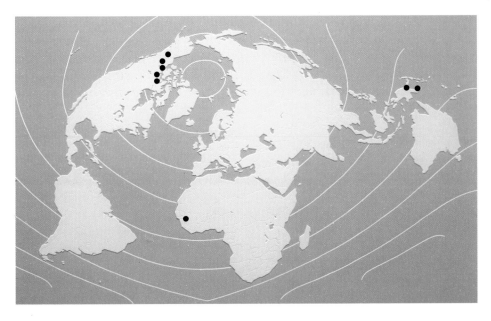

Around the world asthma is on the increase. Australia has the highest incidence but only a handful of places— indicated in black—are completely asthma-free.

In some countries asthma has increased fourfold over the last 30 years and studies show that the increase is real and not just because people are more aware of the condition. The rise is very steep in children. Wheezing illnesses among British teenagers increased by 70 percent between 1974 and 1986.

In Finland, doctors studied military recruits each year between 1920 and 1938. Record-taking resumed after World War II and they discovered that between 1960 and 1990, asthma increased twentyfold. Half the 300-strong population of the island of Tristan da Cunha, a remote island in the South Atlantic between the Cape of Good Hope and Argentina, has asthma.

Although asthma can hit anybody, regardless of race, in New Zealand it is more common in the Maori population. In the United States the biggest increase is among African-Americans living in the inner cities.

Yet in some places it is almost unknown. In northern Canada, only a handful of the indigenous Inuit have been admitted to hospital with asthma symptoms over the past 12 years.

There is no word for asthma in the highlands of Papua New Guinea because the problem is so rare. In the villages of Gambia, the disease is unknown, but it is common in nearby towns. The same is true of the villages and towns of other African countries, including Kenya, Zambia, and Nigeria.

It seems that there is a combination of reasons for the increase in asthma:
- Modern homes encourage the growth of the house dust mite, and children nowadays spend more time indoors than their parents or grandparents did.
- There is more pollution from factories and vehicle exhaust fumes.
- Some doctors think our homes may be too clean. Children need to be exposed to infections in order to build up their immune systems.
- It may be that constant exposure to the hot, dry air usual in centrally heated homes is a factor.

The respiratory system

*M*ost of us never think about breathing until something goes *wrong or we are out of breath from too much exercise. In the process of respiration, the body takes in oxygen—essential for life's vital functions—from the air. Carbon dioxide is produced as a waste product, and this is expelled as we breathe out.*

Exercise can trigger an asthma attack. But you have to find a balance between being protective and allowing your child to participate in normal, enjoyable activities.

When we breathe, air is drawn in through the mouth and nose. It passes through the larynx, or voice box, down the windpipe, or trachea, and into the lungs. The airways are lined with tiny, hairlike cilia. If any particles of dust or dirt enter the system, they are trapped in the mucus lining and the cilia expel them with a waving, escalatorlike motion.

When the trachea reaches the lungs, it divides into two branches, or bronchi, one for each lung. Each bronchus divides into thousands of fine bronchioles, like delicate twigs, each of which ends in a small air sac, called an alveolus. There are around 300 million alveoli in the lungs—each one is surrounded by a mesh of tiny blood vessels. Oxygen passes into the blood through the alveoli, and the oxygenated blood is then sent to the heart, which pumps it around the body.

The waste product of respiration is carbon dioxide, which the body returns to the heart, which in turn pumps it to the lungs. The lungs, having no use for it, expel it. Every day, a total of around 2,000 gallons (10,000 liters) of air moves in and out of the lungs.

The lungs are delicate and encased by the ribs. Each one is further protected by a two-layer membrane, the pleura, which allows the lungs to move in and out easily. Between each rib is thick muscle—intercostal muscle—which expands and contracts with each breath you take. Underneath the lungs is a dome-shaped sheet of muscle, the diaphragm, which rises and falls as you breathe.

The mechanics of breathing

Breathing is involuntary, but, unlike the beating of our heart, we do have some control over it. We can hold our breath, use it to shout, scream, sing, or whistle and breathe from the top of our lungs or from the abdomen.

Breathing itself is not as simple as it might appear. Every time you breathe in the diaphragm flattens and the muscles between the ribs shorten, pulling the rib cage up and out. As the space in the chest cavity expands, the lungs fill with air. When the lungs are full the diaphragm and rib muscles relax and the rib cage contracts, expelling the air.

The rate at which you breathe varies with how much oxygen you need—this information is monitored and controlled by the respiratory center of the brain, the medulla. When you exercise, the body floods with carbon dioxide and needs more oxygen. The medulla signals the lungs to breathe deeper and faster, sometimes as much as 80 times a minute. When you are resting, and carbon dioxide levels return to normal, you take between 13 and 15 breaths a minute.

THE RESPIRATORY SYSTEM

This system takes in air from the atmosphere and transports it to the lungs. In the lungs, oxygen is absorbed into the blood stream and waste carbon dioxide is released to the exterior. The action of intercostal muscles and the diaphragm expand and contract the chest cavity, making the lungs move in and out.

Nasal cavity
The nose filters, warms, and moistens air

Larynx
Contains the vocal cords for voice production

Trachea
Extends down from the larynx toward the lungs

Ribs
Move to expand and contract lungs when breathing in and out

Pleura
A double-layered membrane surrounding the lungs

Diaphragm
Flattens down to breathe in and relaxes to breathe out

Alveoli
Tiny sacs within the lungs where gas exchange takes place between air and blood

Bronchus
Enters lung and divides into smaller bronchioles

The skin system

The skin is the largest organ of the body and protects the internal organs from the environment. It helps regulate body temperature, can repair itself when damaged, and is the first line of defense against harmful microorganisms.

No material made by humans is as resilient and hard-wearing as the skin. It protects us from heat and cold, is waterproof, stretches or shrinks if we put on or lose weight, and flushes when we are nervous.

The skin is also the first thing that people see when they look at us, so it is more than just a protective layer. We want it to be clear and blemish-free and anything that disfigures it causes emotional as well as physical distress. Skin conditions, such as psoriasis or eczema, can destroy a person's self-confidence and affect personal and professional relationships.

Structure of the skin

Skin is made of two layers—a thin outer layer, called the epidermis, and a thick inner layer, the dermis. Below this is a layer of tissue containing fat.

The epidermis is made up of layers of flat cells. It is very thick on the soles of the feet, palms, and knees, and thinnest on the eyelids. The lowest layers of the epidermis contain the mother, or germinating, cells that move up to the surface, where they flatten, die, and are shed—a process that takes about four weeks.

The dermis consists of collagens (a protein) and contains sweat glands, blood vessels, nerves, and hair follicles. The

THE SKIN

The main layers of the skin are the epidermis and the dermis. The fatty inner subcutaneous tissue lies below the dermis. The dermis contains blood vessels, hair follicles, nerves, sweat glands, and sebaceous glands that lubricate the hair and outer surface of the skin.

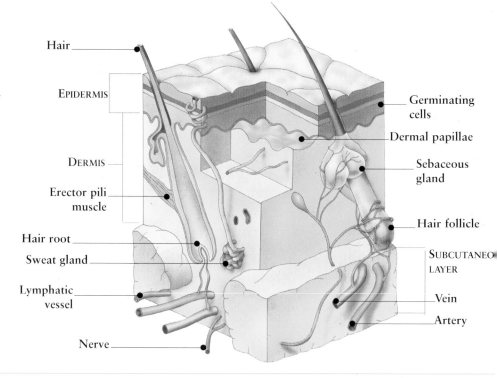

Hair

EPIDERMIS

DERMIS

Erector pili muscle

Hair root

Sweat gland

Lymphatic vessel

Nerve

Germinating cells

Dermal papillae

Sebaceous gland

Hair follicle

SUBCUTANEO LAYER

Vein

Artery

sweat glands regulate body temperature, while the sebaceous glands produce grease and open into the hair follicles.

Skin becomes drier and loses its elasticity as we get older. It begins to look weather-beaten and can be damaged by too much sunlight, heat, or cold.

Skin allergies

In an allergic reaction, your immune system thinks that a substance, which causes most people no harm, is a threat to your body.

• **Urticaria**, also known as nettle rash or hives, takes the form of itchy raised areas, or wheals, on the skin. They are usually pale in the middle and red around the edges and can affect a fifth of us at any one time. Urticaria is the result of touching or eating something to which you are allergic. It can erupt after seconds and normally lasts a few hours.

• **Angioedema** is a severe reaction in which your face, eyelids, and throat swell. It can also hamper your breathing. The outbreaks on the skin resemble those of urticaria, but originate in lower levels of the skin. Though angioedema can be painful, it does not itch.

• **Contact dermatitis** is a condition in which the skin becomes inflamed and develops itchy red patches after contact with a particular substance. The chief culprits are detergents, some of which may be left in washed clothes, nickel (from watch straps, eye-glass frames, and jewelry), cosmetics, some plants (notably primula and poison ivy), chemicals, particularly those in rubber, and preservatives in creams and paints.

• **Eczema** may be another form of contact dermatitis, but it may also be caused by something you've eaten, by stress or by something in the environment. Neither

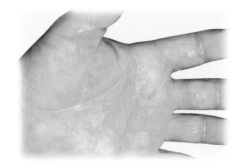

dermatitis nor eczema is infectious. Around one in 20 people has eczema.

What eczema looks and feels like varies from person to person, but most have dry patches of skin that crack, redden, and sometimes bleed. You may have small watery blisters. It may feel hot, itchy, and bubbling. If you scratch a patch of eczema, the skin becomes thick and leathery. But it does not scar and once the eczema clears up it will look as good as new, though it will need to be kept well moisturized.

Types of eczema

Atopic eczema (defined as a hereditary tendency to be hypersensitive to certain allergens) can affect anyone from the age of three months, and is most common in children. It often starts on the face and spreads to the wrists, the insides of the elbows, and the backs of the knees. At its worst it may cover the whole body.

Other forms of eczema include varicose, or stasis, eczema, which develops in places where there are varicose veins. It is usually caused by poor circulation; it can also be inherited. Nummular eczema usually affects adults and looks a bit like ringworm, with circular, itchy scaling patches. No one knows what causes it.

Find out more

Tests for allergies	60
Treatments for the skin	70
Chinese herbal medicine	112

Eczema causes itching and a red rash. The small blisters exude a watery fluid and the skin becomes crusty and flakes.

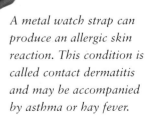

A metal watch strap can produce an allergic skin reaction. This condition is called contact dermatitis and may be accompanied by asthma or hay fever.

The digestive system

*L**ike a complicated chemical factory, the digestive system breaks down the food you eat into its usable nutrients. These are eventually absorbed into the blood and lymph, which transport them throughout the body.***

The gut is about 30 ft (9 m) long and stretches from mouth to anus. It divides into the mouth, gullet (esophagus), stomach, small intestine, large intestine or colon, rectum (bowel), and anus. When everything is working normally, the digestive system is a highly efficient food-absorption and waste-disposal system, sending messages to your brain that tell you when to eat, what to eat, and when to expel waste products.

Each section has a particular function and it sparks into action automatically. Just the thought of food, let alone the sight or smell of it, releases saliva into the mouth in anticipation. Digestion usually takes around 24 hours, but it can take up to three days.

The start of the process

In your mouth, chewing and saliva break food down into a paste ball, or bolus, which passes down the esophagus into your stomach as you swallow. Food is pushed down by powerful muscular contractions called peristalsis and these strong waves occur throughout the gut.

The stomach is a muscular bag shaped like a fat "J." It is just below the diaphragm and can expand to hold about 2½ pints (1.5 liters). Food is worked on and broken down by the mixing and churning of the stomach and by acid secreted by the lining as well as digestive enzymes, such as pepsin. The acid dissolves the food and kills most bacteria. The stomach empties in two to six hours.

Small intestine

The broken-down food, now in the form of a soupy liquid, moves into the next section of the gut, a C-shaped tube about 10 in (25 cm) long that forms the first part of the small intestine.

The gallbladder and pancreatic duct deposit a cocktail of digestive enzymes into this section of the small intestine. This works on the food, breaking down carbohydrates, fats, and proteins.

The food then moves through the rest of the small intestine, which is about 20 ft (6 m) long. Nutrients, minerals, and water are absorbed through the walls and into the blood stream in a process that takes between three and five hours. The inner wall of the small intestine is covered with tiny structures called villi that create a huge surface area through which nutrients can be absorbed.

Colon and rectum

The large intestine, or colon, is about 5 ft (1.5 m) long. Its main function is to absorb any remaining salt and water from the digested food. It contains a myriad of bacteria that prepare waste material for elimination. Up to 1¾ pints (1 liter) of water is absorbed in the colon so that the contents are a semisolid mass. What remains of your meal spends between 12 and 48 hours in the colon.

Waste matter then passes through to the rectum, which acts as a storage container. When the rectum is full, it triggers an elimination reflex and feces leave the body through the anus.

Tongue
Food is rolled into a lump, ready for swallowing

Salivary glands
Secrete enzymes that break down starch

Mouth
Food is chewed to soften it and break it down

Epiglottis
Cartilaginous flap that stops food from entering the trachea during swallowing

Esophagus
Waves of muscular action carry food down the esophagus and into the stomach

Liver
Makes bile, which has a detergent action, breaking fat down into tiny globules

Stomach
Food is churned, digested, and stored for about six hours

Gallbladder
Stores bile until needed for digestion

Pancreas
Releases digestive enzymes that break down starch, fat, and protein

Small intestine
Principal site for the absorption of nutrients

Appendix
Has no known function in humans

Rectum
Muscular tube that expels digestive waste as feces through the anus

Colon
Water is absorbed and bowel contents solidify

The digestive system

For most people, peanuts are totally harmless. But for the unfortunate few who have a peanut allergy, they can cause a violent and potentially dangerous reaction.

Even foods that are usually part of a healthy diet can cause an adverse reaction. They include fish and shellfish, legumes, wheat, sugar, strawberries, and citrus fruits.

Food allergies

There is a big difference between a food allergy and food intolerance. An allergy, such as the one some people have to peanuts, causes the immune system—the body's defense mechanism against bacteria, viruses, and any other intruder—to leap into action. One person in six has a food allergy. Sometimes a person is born allergic to something; often an allergy may develop.

Foods such as papaya, shellfish, and strawberries, which to anyone else would be totally harmless, can make a person who is allergic to them extremely ill because of this exaggerated immune response. The skin may erupt into a rash, wheeziness may occur, the face may swell, and the stomach may become upset.

In severe cases of food allergy, the person may collapse and, without an injection of epinephrine, could die. This serious condition is called anaphylactic shock (see p. 33 for first aid).

Food intolerance

When you have an adverse reaction to a particular food, but there is no evidence that your immune system has gone into overdrive, nor is your life in danger, this is food intolerance. Intolerances are usually caused because your body does not produce enough of a particular enzyme to digest that substance properly.

Gluten

Apart from triggering asthma, hay fever, and eczema, allergies can also cause other problems. These include celiac disease (or celiac sprue), an intestinal disorder brought on by gluten, found in wheat; inflammatory bowel disease; irritable bowel syndrome; hyperactivity in children; and other conditions, such as panic attacks, tiredness, mild depression, headaches, and excess mucus.

Some people with gluten sensitivity develop an itchy rash with small raised patches and blisters. These often occur on the elbows, buttocks, and knees, although they can affect any area of the skin.

If you have dermatitis herpetiformis—literally "reptilelike skin inflammation"—your digestion may be unaffected, but you may feel slightly bloated and have more bowel motions than normal. The condition is cured by eliminating gluten from your diet.

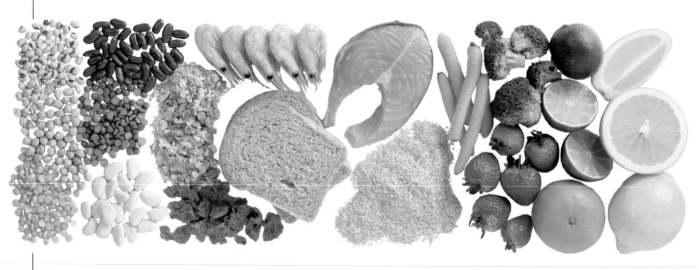

BAD REACTION TO FOOD?

If you react badly to a food it could be due to one of the following:
• A genuine food allergy, where your body's immune system mistakenly thinks it is under attack
• Food poisoning caused by bacterially contaminated food
• Food sensitivity that triggers a medical condition, such as a migraine. You may find that eating chocolate or drinking red wine starts off such a headache
• Food intolerance, where your body has difficulty in processing a particular food.

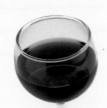

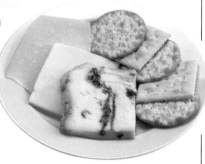

Symptoms of food allergy

The symptoms may develop the moment you come into contact with the food. Your tongue and lips may tingle, and the lips and inside of your mouth may swell up. You may have abdominal cramps, feel nauseous, or vomit.

You could also experience an allergic reaction on your skin, which may erupt into a rash or urticaria or angioedema. Other signs of an allergy are chest symptoms, such as wheezing and coughing. The food could also trigger an asthma attack or make a skin condition, such as eczema, flare up.

Symptoms of food intolerance

The symptoms of food intolerance are not as violent as those associated with food allergy. Many may be chronic, or long-standing. You may have headaches and migraines or feel tired and depressed. If your child is intolerant of certain foods he or she may become hyperactive.

You may suffer from recurrent canker sores, aching muscles, and have gut disorders, such as irritable bowel syndrome, or rheumatoid arthritis.

Foods that can cause allergy and intolerance

A person can be allergic to or intolerant of any food—eggs, cheese, citrus fruit, sugar, cabbage, pork, the list is endless. Many people quite happily eat foods, such as alcohol and caffeine, found in tea and coffee, that their bodies do not really like in large quantities, but without any apparent ill effects. Some people pride themselves on tolerating foods, such as the hottest of curries, which other people would shy away from, yet turn their noses up at foods that rarely—if ever—make people sick, such as tapioca, broccoli, melons, and rice. It all depends on the individual.

Common culprits

The following foods are those that most commonly cause an adverse reaction:
• Cow's milk and dairy products
• Nuts
• Wheat
• Food additives
• Alcohol
• Shellfish.

Sensitivity to red wine or dairy products such as cheese can lead to a migraine or other generalized aches and pains.

The immune system

This is the body's protective system and it works like a highly trained army fighting off invaders, such as bacteria and viruses, and foreign bodies, such as a splinter or insect venom. This army is made up of different cells, each with its own job to

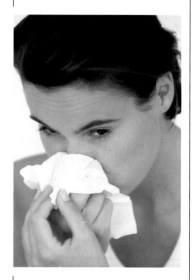

When an allergen triggers the immune system's defenses, the body releases histamine, causing the classic allergy symptoms of swollen, watery, and itchy nose, eyes, and sinuses.

The body's first line of defense includes the skin, tonsils, the hair in your nose, and mucus in your nostrils and lungs. Stomach acid destroys the most harmful microorganisms. Enzymes in saliva and tears also kill bacteria.

If an invader does manage to make it past these defenses, however, the "ground troops" go to war. These are divided into white blood cells, or B cells, which are made in the bone marrow, and T cells, also made in the bone marrow, and which may mature in the lymph glands.

B cells produce chemicals called antibodies or immunoglobulin. There are five types of antibody—one group plays an important part in allergies. They lock on to the surface of foreign substances, or antigens, such as bacteria, and so help destroy them. Once the invading cells have been covered in antibodies they are easy prey for the T cells, which move in for the kill.

Usually this system works well, protecting us from most diseases. But it relies on the B cells correctly recognizing an invader and going to work. Sometimes it works when we would prefer that it did not—by attacking a transplanted organ that it sees as foreign, for example.

The immune system is programmed to remember invaders and will muster its forces at the slightest hint of a threat. Scientists can even "trick" the immune system into "remembering" invaders, such as smallpox, that it hasn't actually encountered by exposing it to traces of a similar virus, such as cowpox.

System failure

Diseases that result from the immune system's failure to function properly range from herpes and fungal infections to AIDS. Sometimes, the immune system turns on itself and damages the body in the same way that troops accidentally fire on their allies. It attacks its own tissues as if they were foreign substances. This "friendly fire" is responsible for diabetes, the skin-lightening disease known as vitiligo, and some forms of anemia.

The allergic reaction

B cells make the "allergy" antibody immunoglobulin E, or IgE (pronounced as the letters i, g, e). IgE is normally produced in response to parasites, such as ringworm and liver fluke, so if you live in the developed world you will not normally have much of this antibody in your blood. However, if you live in a developing country, you may have high levels of IgE.

If you suffer from asthma or allergies you will have a high level of IgE in your blood because you have an oversensitive immune system that goes into action against substances that most people's immune systems regard as harmless, such as a peanut or the droppings of the house dust mite. This is what is known as an allergic reaction and the substance that causes it is an allergen.

When the allergen, which may be dog hairs, pollen, or dust mite droppings, enters the body, it is immediately but mistakenly identified by the immune

INSIDE THE AIRWAYS

The inner surface of the windpipe is covered with tiny hairlike cilia. Particles entering from the air outside are trapped in the mucus lining and pushed out by the beating action of the cilia. In this colored scanning electron micrograph, the cilia are green, trapped pollen grains are orange, and dust particles brown.

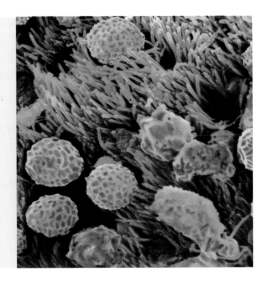

system as a dangerous substance—so the immune system produces a flood of protective IgE antibodies.

These antibodies fix themselves by their stem onto special cells called mast cells, present in the skin, stomach lining, lungs, and upper airways. The mast cells then release various chemicals, the main ones being histamine and leukotrienes, which are responsible for the allergic reaction. Histamine causes the blood vessels to widen, fluid to leak from the tissues, and the muscles to go into spasm. Histamines also attract other cells, which cause further damage and inflammation.

These chemicals produce all the classic allergy systems—itchy red skin, sneezing, watery eyes, narrowing of the airways, vomiting and diarrhea—and, in extreme cases, anaphylactic shock.

Allergies result from exposure to a substance—often when we are babies, sometimes even in the womb—and this leads to the production of IgE. This is called sensitization and the allergic reaction happens only on the second or even third exposure. Babies born in the pollen season are therefore more likely to develop hay fever than those born in winter. Similarly, a child exposed to high levels of the house dust mite before the age of one—by living in a house with thick carpets, upholstery, and drapes—is more likely to develop asthma in childhood.

FOREIGN BODIES

The immune system's function is to repel "invaders" such as the Adeno viruses shown in red here. These viruses infect the upper respiratory tract, producing symptoms similar to those of the common cold.

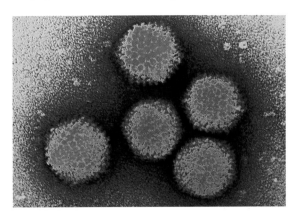

Asthma and your airways

Your lungs can usually cope with microscopic invaders. A quick cough or sneeze and they're instantly expelled. But when you have asthma, your immune response will leap into action if you breathe in any substance to which you are allergic.

The normal airway, or bronchus, is lined with a fine protective layer—the mucosa or epithelium. Some cells in this layer produce fluid or mucus, while others pass these secretions up the bronchial tubes to the mouth by moving tiny hairlike cells, or cilia, which coat the surface of these cells. The mucus is then swallowed, to be sterilized by the acid in the stomach, or expelled by coughing. Cilia are destroyed by smoking, which is why so many smokers develop a phlegmy cough.

Below the mucosa is the submucosa, which in turn encases a spiral sheet of muscle. This muscle can tighten suddenly to protect the air sacs when you inhale something you shouldn't, such as water.

Asthma is caused when the airways become inflamed to such an extent that some are even blocked. This inflammation may be triggered by inhaling an allergen, such as pollen. If you breathe in an allergen it penetrates deep into your lungs and lodges in the tiny air sacs, called alveoli. The immune system recognizes the allergen as an invader—even though it is not—and sends out antibodies, setting off an allergic reaction.

Inflammation is the body's way of dealing with infection and usually it is short-lived. However, in asthma the inflammation of the airways can last for several hours. This increases the mucus in the lungs and can leave the bronchi sensitive, often for a number of days.

If you have attack after attack the inflammation does not have the chance to calm down; instead the condition develops

CASE HISTORY

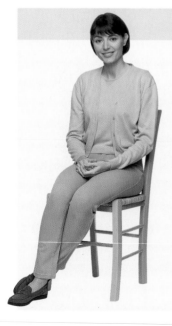

Miranda, 35, developed asthma when she was 25. "I'd always had colds and chesty coughs but never realized that it would lead to asthma. But after three years working as a teacher, my health deteriorated rapidly and I had to learn to cope with severe asthma. I really enjoyed teaching, but my asthma interfered with it to the point where I had to face the fact that I could no longer work."

Miranda was having attacks almost every day. "You just can't get enough air down to keep the body going. It's like a

vice around your chest. Imagine what it's like wearing a Victorian corset and having to have yourself laced up really tight and that's what it feels like. You feel short of breath and you're trying to breathe in, but you can't take in any more air because it hurts so much.

"Once I've had my medication I'm back to normal within 10 minutes, but if I have a really bad attack, it can take days before I feel right. A couple of times I was concerned that I might not survive. Those who do not suffer have no idea how frightening an attack can be."

into a chronic, or long-term, illness. In severe cases of asthma the airways thicken and mucus plugs block the bronchi, even when you are not having an attack. It is also likely that even moderately affected asthmatics have some degree of inflammation between attacks.

An acute asthma attack

Inflammation in the airways causes them to narrow in one of three ways: they may flood with mucus, the inner lining of the bronchi may swell, or the spiral muscles in the bronchi may constrict—or in the worst cases a combination of all three. This leads to the characteristic wheezing as you struggle to breathe. Your chest will feel tight, you may cough up phlegm, and you will be short of breath. In an acute attack, it will be difficult to breathe in, and you will feel as though someone is suffocating you.

Classic symptoms of an asthma attack include the following:

- Difficulty in breathing accompanied by loud wheezing, especially when breathing out.
- Hyperventilation—that is, breathing more rapidly than normal.
- Pushed out chest and difficulty in speaking.
- A blue tinge to the face, especially around the lips and mouth—a sign that you are not getting enough oxygen.
- Racing pulse and sweating.

A severe asthma attack is a medical emergency and needs to be treated by a doctor and in a hospital. The racing pulse could just mean that you are scared or it could be caused by the bronchodilator (the medication you are likely to administer yourself by means of a puffer) which stimulates the release of epinephrine.

Find out more

Respiratory system	18
Drugs for asthma	64
Emergency treatment	154

In an asthma attack, make sure the sufferer uses reliever medication immediately; if that has no effect within 5–10 minutes, dial 911; continue with the medication until help arrives.

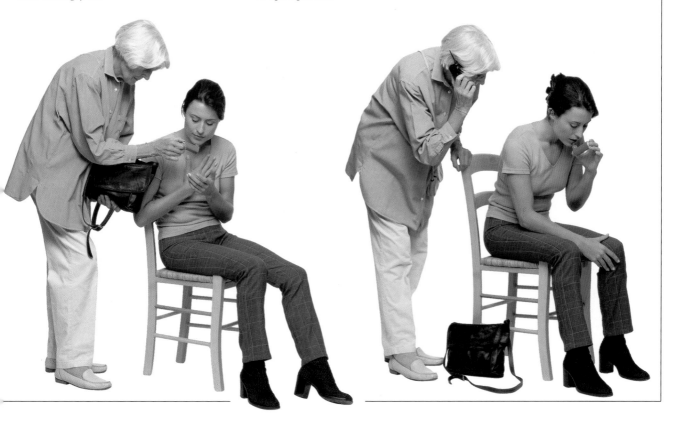

Extreme allergic reactions

*A*naphylaxis, or anaphylactic shock, is a severe allergic *reaction in which the whole body is affected, usually within minutes of coming into contact with an allergen. It leads to acute breathing difficulties and often causes a widespread rash.*

Breastfeeding generally reduces the incidence of asthma. Nevertheless, there is a small but significant risk that your baby can acquire an allergic sensitivity through breast milk. To be on the safe side, do not eat too many nuts when you are breastfeeding.

Anaphylactic shock can cause headache, itchy skin, stomach cramps, nausea and vomiting, coughing and sneezing, difficulty in breathing, and even convulsions and loss of consciousness. Anything can set off this extreme reaction, but the usual culprits are bee and wasp stings, or eating peanuts and other nuts. Occasionally sesame seeds, natural latex (rubber), fish, shellfish, fresh fruit, penicillin or any drug or injection, dairy products, and eggs can also cause anaphylactic shock.

Warning: In all cases of anaphylactic shock, it is essential to administer first aid immediately, while waiting for medical assistance. An epinephrine injection can be a life-saver (see p.33).

Peanut allergy

As many as one in 200 people may be allergic to peanuts and most schools have one or two children with a peanut allergy. It seems to be on the increase and this is believed to be because more people eat peanuts as a snack and more parents give their babies foods containing peanuts.

It is difficult to protect yourself if you have anaphylaxis, and you have to be very careful about what you eat. Peanuts, for instance, turn up unexpectedly in all kinds of foods, not just the more obvious ones like peanut butter. Traces of nuts can be found in chocolate bars, ready-made supermarket meals, airline meals, cakes, and desserts.

In October 1993, a 17-year-old girl died after eating a slice of lemon meringue pie served to her in the restaurant of a department store. It contained peanuts, to which she was fatally allergic. In another incident, a 19-year-old artist died of an allergic reaction to walnuts, which were in a homemade sherry trifle.

Babies can become sensitized to allergens through breast milk and it is wise to avoid eating large quantities of peanuts, almonds, brazil nuts, and walnuts if you are breastfeeding,

HUMAN AIR FILTER

Hairlike cilia line the surface of all the body's cells, beating rhythmically to move the cell or the medium that surrounds it. In among the cilia of the trachea are so-called goblet cells. These produce mucus, which in addition to trapping particles from inhaled air, removes unwanted gases such as ozone and sulfur dioxide. Excess mucus production can cause asthma. In this false color scanning electron micrograph, goblet cells appear dark orange and the cilia are yellow.

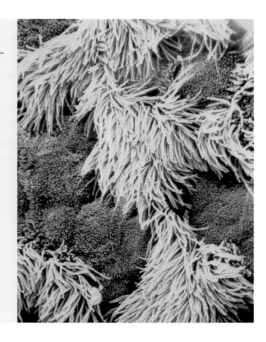

though small quantities will do no harm. Some nipple lotions even contain peanut oil, and formula milk in the 1970s and 1980s contained peanut oil which could sensitize the baby (most manufacturers have now removed it). Research has shown that mothers may sensitize their babies to peanuts before birth as particles of peanut protein eaten by the mother pass through the placenta to the baby.

Unrefined peanut oil can bring on a severe reaction, but researchers have found that refined peanut oil will not cause allergic reactions in most people allergic to peanuts, and if anyone does suffer a reaction it is likely to be mild because the refining process removes the peanut protein. The oilseed industry is currently setting up a code of practice to ensure that unrefined peanut oil will always be declared on the label.

If you suffer a peanut allergy it is wise to avoid skin preparations, such as eczema creams, that contain peanut oil.

Some scientists think there may be a link between these creams and peanut allergies in children. If you are breastfeeding, avoid nipple lotions that contain peanut oil.

Stings and bites

The venom of snakes and insects is another trigger for anaphylactic shock. The incidence of snake bites is not great, and few people die as a result of being bitten. However, every year, a handful of people in most countries will die as a result of a severe allergic reaction to a bee, wasp, or hornet sting. In addition, some "mystery" deaths in people over 40, thought to be caused by heart attacks, may have been caused by a sting.

Most of us are frightened of being stung—it's a nasty, painful experience and causes the skin around the sting site to swell. But people who are allergic to bees and wasps live in fear of being stung. If they do not receive an epinephrine injection, the sting could be fatal.

Extreme allergic reactions

Bee stings

Honeybees are not aggressive insects and will attack only if they think their colony is under threat. Bumble bees are not aggressive either, but they will sting if they are trodden on. So if you have an allergy to bee stings, don't walk around barefoot in the grass.

When a bee stings you, it leaves its stinger, with the venom sac attached, in its victim. Because it takes a few minutes for all the venom to seep in, you should pull the stinger out as fast as you can. Be careful how you remove it, though. If you just try to grab it, you're likely to squeeze in more venom. The best way is to flick it out with a fingernail or knife blade.

Wasp stings

Wasps are extremely bad-tempered insects, particularly in late summer and autumn. Their stinger does not pull away from their body and they can sting again and again. Kitchen garbage cans, outdoor trash cans, and rotting fruit are all fair game for the hungry wasp. So if you are picking fruit, be extremely careful.

You can still find wasps in late autumn and early winter. They are sleepy and less active, but just as dangerous.

How to avoid being stung

If you are allergic to insect stings, take these basic precautions:

• Avoid wearing bright clothing, flowery prints, or black because these seem to attract bees and other insects.

• Wear shoes outside.

• Don't use strong perfumes in summer and be careful with suntan lotions, hair gels, and cosmetics, which can also contain perfume.

• Cover up your arms and legs if you can.

• Use an insect repellent if you are outside for some time, particularly if you're on your own.

• Food attracts insects, so keep food and trash cans covered.

WHAT YOU CAN DO

The treatment for a violent allergic reaction is epinephrine, the "fight or flight" hormone normally released when a person meets danger. It prepares the body to cope with stress. If you know you have such a severe allergy you should always carry an epinephrine "pen," which is often known as an Epi-pen.

This has a spring-loaded concealed needle and is easy to administer either to yourself or to a friend and can be used on children as young as two. If your symptoms are mild, you can use an epinephrine inhaler. But if you have been prescribed both, carry both. It is the injection that will save your life.

If your child has severe allergies, tell the school and make sure there is someone there who knows how to use the Epi-pen. You have to teach your child to be scrupulous about reading food labels, and tell friends and friends' parents about the allergy.

Find out more

| Immune system | 26 |
| Airborne allergens | 42 |

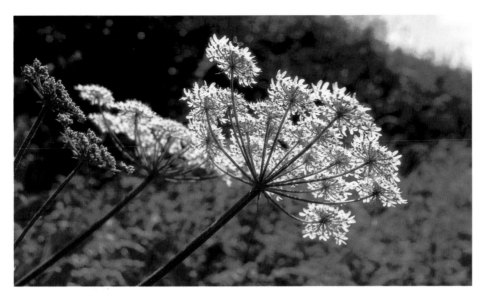

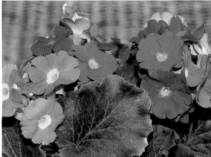

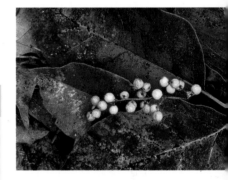

• Wasps slip into food and drinks when you're not looking, so always look at what you're eating and never drink out of a can or bottle.

• Don't try to swat an insect if it flies near you—just move slowly away.
• If an insect lands on you, don't panic. It will usually fly away after a few seconds.

FIRST AID FOR ANAPHYLACTIC SHOCK

ANAPHYLACTIC SHOCK

The immune system goes into overdrive, and within seconds of exposure to a foreign body, any of the following symptoms may occur:

• Itching or a strange metallic taste in the mouth
• Swelling of the throat and tongue, creating the risk of suffocation
• Difficulty in breathing because of severe asthma or a swollen throat
• Flushing of the skin
• Cramps and nausea
• Increased heart rate
• A sudden feeling of weakness because your blood pressure has dropped dramatically
• Urticaria anywhere on the body
• Collapse and unconsciousness

EMERGENCY MEASURES
• Loosen the victim's clothing at the neck and the waist
• Check that the airways are open. Support the victim in a position that allows him or her to breathe easily
• If the victim starts to vomit, turn the head to one side so that the airways do not become blocked
• Check whether the chest is rising and, with your ear next to their mouth, listen and feel for breath
• Check for a pulse by gently pressing two fingers at the side of the neck, next to the Adam's apple
• If the victim was stung by an insect, remove the stinger carefully
• Apply emergency medication, if the victim carries any (see box opposite)

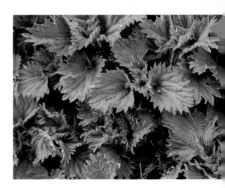

Plants that cause allergic reactions include hogweed (top left), primula (top), poison ivy (middle), and nettle (bottom).

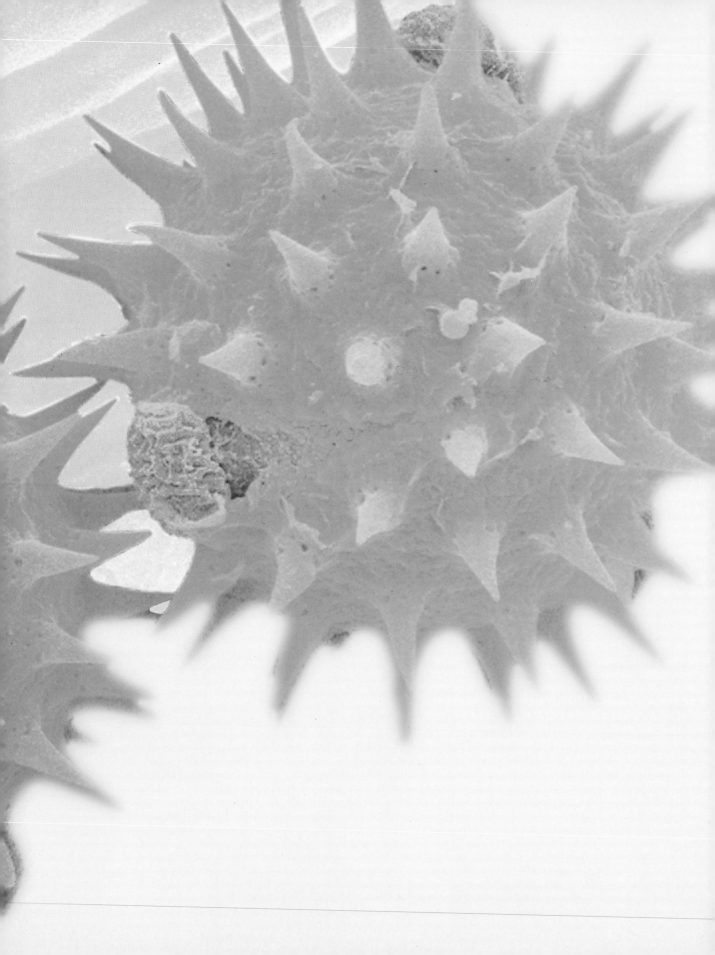

2

CAUSES AND SOLUTIONS

A trigger is something that sparks off an allergy or asthma attack. It is a substance that sets a series of physical changes in motion that leads to the telltale wheezing and breathlessness of an asthmatic, the sneezing and streaming eyes of a hay fever sufferer, and the itchy skin rashes of someone with eczema. Even if you have an inherited weakness—if asthma and allergies seem to run in your family—a trigger is still needed to make the "seed" that has been laid down in your genes flourish and grow.

For most people, regular exercise can make a useful contribution to good health. But if carried out to excess, it may provoke an asthma attack. Consult your doctor before following an exercise program and be aware of your own limits. You can also take steps to keep your environment as free of potential triggers as possible.

Allergy triggers

T*he triggers of asthma and allergies include pollution, exercise, stress and emotion, physical triggers, occupational triggers, the weather, and food and drug allergies.*

Indoor pollution

The chief culprit indoors is the house dust mite—or more specifically, its droppings. The house dust mite is a member of the spider family. It looks like an ugly monster in blown-up photographs, but in fact it is so small it cannot be seen by the naked eye. It loves carpets, curtains, bedding, soft toys, and upholstered furniture, and thrives when there is a little bit of warm moisture in the air.

Household pets, particularly cats, are a potent allergen. Dogs, too, can trigger an attack, and some people report that hamsters, gerbils, horses, guinea pigs, rats, and mice can also bring on coughing, wheezing, and breathlessness.

In the past, houses were drafty, with the wind whistling through cracks in the window frames, gaps under the doors, and down the chimney. One study showed that in such a house the air in a room changed seven times a hour. Now we have insulation and sealed doors and windows and the air changes about once an hour. Pollutants hang in the air and dust, nitrogen dioxide (NO_2) fumes from unventilated gas stoves, cigarettes, and chemicals from perfume and cleaning fluids—all of which are potent triggers—have nowhere to escape. Molds also thrive indoors, particularly in older houses, which may be damp, and in poorly ventilated modern homes.

Outdoor pollution

Outside, a cocktail of pollutants can trigger asthma and allergies. Power plants pump out sulfur dioxide (SO_2), produced when coal is burned, and both diesel and nondiesel vehicles have exhaust emissions thick with NO_2.

Hanging in a thick layer in some cities in summer is ozone, part of a pattern of air pollution known as photochemical smog. These smogs are caused by a chemical reaction in the air near the earth's surface brought on by bright sunlight. When these gases react with water vapor, acid air results. Studies show that people living near roads are more likely to suffer from asthma and allergies than those who live farther away.

In certain weather conditions, the emissions from vehicles, power plants, and factories combine to form a toxic mixture in the pall of smog that hangs over some large cities.

Spores from grass, tree, and plant pollen can trigger hay fever and other allergies, as can molds. Both spores and molds are abundant in composters, around rotting leaves, just before a thunderstorm, and near fields in the summer and the fall.

The weather

Thunderstorms have the effect of making pollen burst open and release small starch granules, which can be bad news for asthmatics. On the evening of June 24, 1995, 84 hospitals in southeastern England were filled with nearly 1,000 people complaining of breathing difficulties. As a result, many hospitals ran out of medication.

The outbreak, which affected hay fever rather than asthma sufferers, was caused by a mesoscale convector system. This series of small thunderstorms raced up the English Channel, joined together, clipped northwestern France, headed up over southern England, and exited over the northeast. It was a rare type of storm, seen only once every three or four years.

The storm acted like a giant vacuum cleaner—sucking up the pollutants, mixing them in the atmosphere, and charging them, which made them stick to people's lungs. It then dumped the pollutants back on the ground in concentrated pockets.

It was these dumped particles, possibly burst pollen grains, that triggered the outbreak. Such was the impact of the storm that scientists in Spain, Italy, Austria, Germany, and Switzerland have joined forces to investigate the link between asthma, allergies and the weather. They hope, ultimately, to develop a comprehensive European asthma forecast service. ▶

You can't be allergic to the weather, but it can have a powerful influence. Storms can stir up allergenic particles in the atmosphere and deposit them at ground level, causing mass outbreaks of asthma.

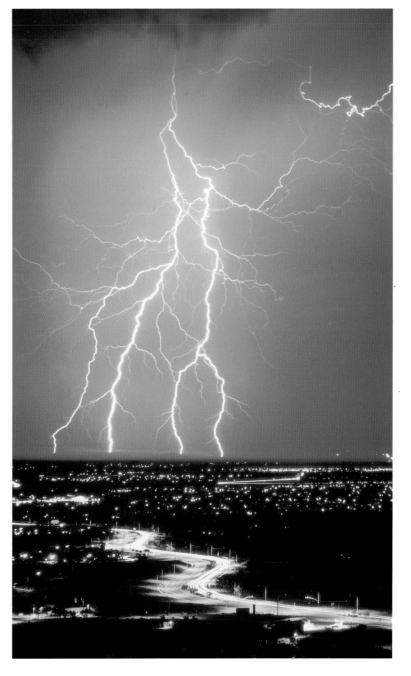

Allergy triggers

Exercise

Most asthma sufferers find that vigorous exercise can trigger an attack. Instead of their breathing calming down naturally as they relax after exercise, some people find they cannot get their breath back. This is most likely to happen when the weather is cold and dry.

This does not mean that you should not exercise at all. Carried out regularly and in moderation, and possibly with advice from your doctor, exercise can certainly improve your well-being. Many experts say that swimming is the best exercise for asthmatics.

Stress and emotion

Fear, excitement, falling in love—all these strong emotions can literally "take your breath away." Researchers now think that a person's emotional life can have an impact on asthma and allergies. There is no evidence that stress causes asthma, but it has been shown to make it worse.

Some doctors think there is an "asthma personality." These people, they say, are irritable, easily angered, always complaining, and obsessive. They suppress their emotions and bottle things up. Some children have been known to bring on an asthma attack by coughing or crying and this is often a way in which they can manipulate their parents.

Other doctors think there is no such thing as an asthma personality. They believe that if people with asthma are a bit anxious this is understandable because they are afraid of an attack.

Physical triggers

Colds and viral infections can trigger an asthma attack—this is particularly common in children. It is a vicious circle, because as the lungs become scarred a

person is more prone to catch a cold. Doctors sometimes prescribe antibiotics to stop asthma from worsening, but these drugs are effective only against infections caused by bacteria, not viruses.

Occupational triggers

If your asthma began after you started a new job or when the conditions of your work changed, you may have occupational asthma. It is easy to identify—it is worst when you are at work and disappears on the weekend and during vacations.

Drug allergies

Most drugs have side effects and if you have asthma or an allergy you must be careful that the medication you take for other conditions—even for a cold—does not make you more vulnerable to an attack. Aspirin and other nonsteroidal anti-inflammatory drugs (NSAIDs), both of which can be bought over the counter, can trigger an attack.

Poverty

Some people believe that asthma, hay fever, and other allergies are more common in educated, professional groups. Research has borne this out—a recent American study found that hay fever was more common among those with high incomes, and in Switzerland hay fever is three times more common among professionals than among manual workers. But British researchers, however, have found that the poorer you are, the more likely you are to have asthma. Indeed, people on low incomes, in poorly paid employment, or unemployed and living in cold, damp homes are twice as likely to develop asthma than those in higher-paid employment, with more a comfortable lifestyle.

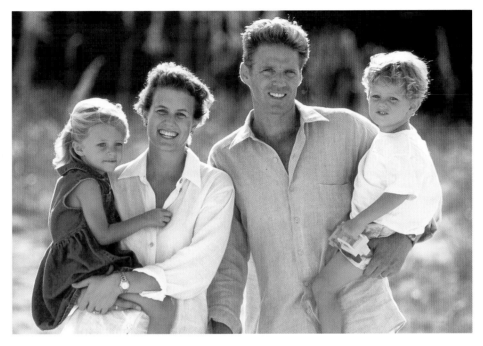

Scientists have yet to find direct genetic evidence, but it is clear that the tendency to have allergies runs in families. Family members may be sensitive to different allergens.

Can you inherit asthma and allergies?

Some people sail through life seemingly devoid of an allergic response. They can eat anything, sit in a field of freshly mown grass without so much as a sniffle, live in dusty old houses, and be surrounded by pets. But it is quite a different story for others—it is almost as if they were born with allergies.

There is a good deal of truth in this for there is little doubt that both asthma and allergies run in families. If you have asthma or allergies, look closely at your family and you'll probably come up with a grandparent or an uncle with asthma, cousins with hay fever or eczema allergies, or an aunt with food allergies. If your mother or father has asthma you could develop it too. Surveys show that in about half of a group of patients with allergies such as eczema, hay fever, urticaria, and asthma, there was a family history of those conditions.

If you have allergic asthma, you probably have a family history of allergic conditions, such as asthma, hay fever, and eczema, all of which are lumped under the heading of atopy. Usually it follows a pattern. In some families, most members will have hay fever; in others it will be asthma; and so on.

Being atopic means that you may have inherited a tendency to have an allergy, though you might not inherit the actual allergy itself. Just because your mother is allergic to cats does not mean you will have exactly the same allergy. You may, for instance, have hay fever or food intolerances instead.

When you inherit some characteristic, whether it's blue eyes and blond hair or a tendency to develop an illness, this instruction for your body to develop in a certain way is laid down in your genes. Scientists now believe that there may be many genes that make you susceptible to allergies.

Allergens in the home

*Y*ou may think that you keep your home impeccably clean. *But there will always be some potential trigger for allergies lurking in carpets and pillows or floating invisibly in the air.*

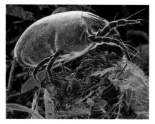

The house dust mite is an unwelcome guest in every home. Its favorite hiding places include carpets, bedding, and furniture.

Dust mites congregate in pillows and mattresses, literally in the millions. If you are an asthma sufferer, take measures to eliminate them.

House dust mites

There are several different types of house dust mite. *Dermatophagoides pteronyssinus* is the most widespread in Europe, while *Dermatophagoides farinae* is the commonest in North America. Whatever the type of mite, they all look much the same.

With its hard scaly shell and menacing pincers, the house dust mite looks truly awesome when magnified. In reality, it is tinier than a pinhead and around two million can live comfortably in one mattress. About 10 percent of the weight of an average pillow is made up of shed skin and house dust mites.

These creatures also live in carpets and soft furnishings such as curtains and sofas.

They burrow into soft toys and cling to clothes, particularly those made of wool. They thrive on humidity and fare particularly well in centrally heated and air-conditioned homes, sealed against the wind and cold. They must have warmth—temperatures around 65–70°F (18–21°C) are ideal. They cannot survive when it is too cold or too hot.

Each mite lives for about 10 weeks and an adult can lay 50–80 eggs in that time. They feed on the skin scales that are shed from the body at a rate of 0.035 oz (1 g) a day. They are aptly named—*derma* is the Greek for "skin" and *phagein* is Greek for "to eat."

It is not the mite itself that causes irritation to the airways but its droppings, or more exactly, a protein that coats the droppings. The droppings are light, and they remain floating in the air. You whip them up into invisible clouds whenever you walk over the carpets. We inhale the clouds and this causes the trouble.

No matter how clean your home, the mite will always be there, as they will be

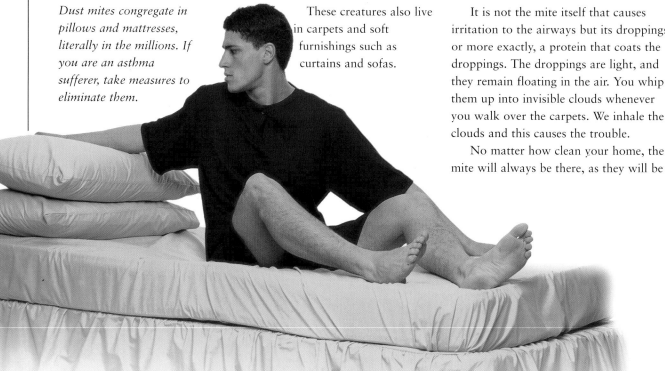

MOLDS AND SPORES

Among the many common triggers of allergies are molds and spores. They thrive in damp houses, in potting compost, and in the moist atmosphere of a greenhouse. This color scanning electron micrograph shows the fruiting body of the common bread mold. The spores form into a cap and then disperse into the air. When the spores land on a piece of bread, they germinate and grow into a mold.

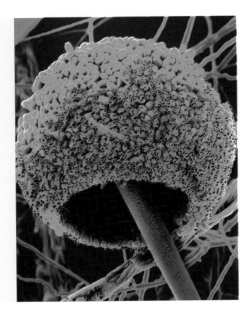

in any building where there is upholstered furniture, including cinemas. They huddle in the seams of chairs, around buttons, and under cushions.

The dust mite has become more important as an asthma trigger because recent research shows that people are spending more time indoors than ever before, watching television or playing computer games.

Molds and spores

When people think of asthma or hay fever, they may think about the house dust mite or pollen, but rarely about molds. Molds belong to a group of living things called fungi, and they reproduce by means of spores. Mushrooms and toadstools are also fungi, but molds are much smaller and colonize rotting vegetation, damp walls, and dead wood. They are the green spots on stale bread and in cheeses such as Roquefort and Stilton.

Molds begin to grow on a slice of bread, for example, because an airborne spore has landed on it. Molds cover everything and there are tens of millions of spores in each cubic yard of air—far more than pollen or house dust mite droppings.

Most spores are harmless and cause no trouble at all, but in the cold, damp countries of the northern hemisphere there are about 20 molds that can trigger allergies and asthma. You can be tested to see if you have an allergy to any particular one at an allergy clinic (see p. 61).

AMALGAM FILLINGS

Many people have teeth filled with amalgam. Though there are gold and white synthetic substitutes, many dentists still fill teeth with this iron-gray metal because it is cheaper and more hard wearing. People in their thirties and upward may have a mouthful of amalgam because dentists filled healthy teeth just to "prevent" them from decaying. Such a practice is now rare.

Some experts believe that tiny traces of mercury present in the amalgam can leach out and cause a wide range of symptoms— difficulty in concentrating, a poor memory, headaches, and circulatory disorders. These researchers now believe that asthma, eczema, and other allergies may be triggered by dental amalgam.

Airborne allergens

Pollen

The fine dust in a flower that fertilizes other plants of the same type is pollen. It is the male part of the plant, equivalent to an animal's semen, and is carried in the wind or picked up on the legs of foraging bees and butterflies, and finally lands on the stigma, or female part, of the plant.

When pollen blows into the eyes and nose of people with hay fever, it sets off an allergic reaction. The antibodies triggered by this reaction stick to the immune mast cells. This causes the mast cells to release inflammatory chemicals, which lead to hay fever symptoms.

The pollen that causes hay fever or asthma is not from hay at all, but from grasses (also tree and plant pollen) and is at its height in early summer. In northern Europe, grass pollen causes the greatest problem, while in the U.S., ragweed is the most common source of allergens.

Workers at orchards and people living nearby can suffer from hay fever in spring, when the trees are in blossom.

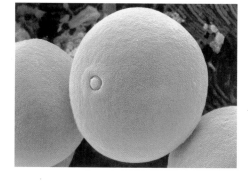

The pollen from cat's tail, also known as timothy grass, is very light and disperses easily in the wind. It is a common trigger of hay fever.

Allergies are not just confined to flower pollen—pollen from hazel, elm, ash, birch, oak, plantain, sorrel, and nettle can also trigger an attack. Similarly, the season is not just confined to the summer months. Pollen from orchards of apples or plums can trigger hay fever among the local population and it is a known fact that florists frequently develop allergies to their products.

In cooler climates, hay fever tends to be a little more common in towns and cities than in rural areas. For example, in Scandinavia it is more common in the towns, and the same is true in other parts of northern Europe and in eastern Europe. Italians are twice as likely to suffer from hay fever if they live in a city rather than the countryside.

But in dry arid countries, the reverse tends to be true. Here plants may grow vigorously but the pollen tends to stay around the farms because there is little wind to blow it into the towns and cities and little or almost no rain to bring it down to earth. In all the countries of Africa, hay fever is virtually unknown, though in India, in contrast, it is common.

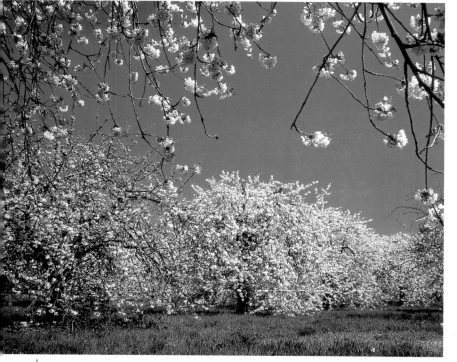

Household pets

No matter how clean the home, or how well it is guarded against dust mites and mold spores, no one who is an asthma sufferer should live in a house with an animal. About half of the people who have asthma are sensitive to allergens produced by animals, mainly cats and dogs. If a baby who has a tendency to inherit allergies is exposed to a cat within the first few months of life then there is an 80 percent chance that he or she will develop an allergy later on.

Cats

These animals are scrupulously clean and spend much of the day grooming themselves. But it is precisely their cleanliness that causes the trouble. As they lick themselves, they flick minute specks of saliva onto their coats. The saliva contains a protein that becomes airborne as it dries. This is the main allergen for those people who are affected and so it does not matter if the cat is long- or short-haired.

Cats produce more allergens than dogs—and so more people are allergic to them—because they clean themselves so much. Most people who have such an allergy know about it the moment a cat jumps on their lap—and cats invariably seem to be attracted to people who do not like them. But you don't have to come into direct physical contact with the cat, nor does there even have to be a cat in the house. Cat salivary protein has been found in houses where no cat has set a paw for many years.

Salivary protein is the main allergen, but fur and animal skin scales—the mixture is called dander—can also cause symptoms, mainly because they too carry salivary protein.

Dogs

Although they are less likely to cause an allergic reaction than cats, dogs can be the cause of asthma, rhinitis, and eczema. As well as salivary protein in the dander, dogs also excrete allergens in their feces and urine.

Feathered friends?

Animals with fur and hair are not the only pets that can cause allergic reactions. Birds can also cause allergies, and owners of parrots, canaries, budgies, and other birds may become allergic to their droppings and feathers. This causes a condition known as alveolitis or bird-fancier's lung, in which an allergic reaction causes the alveoli (air sacs) in the lungs to become inflamed.

Cockroaches

In many hot countries in particular, there are reports of cockroach allergy. In the U.S. up to 30 percent of people with allergies, particularly children living in inner-city areas, are sensitive to the feces and skin particles of cockroaches.

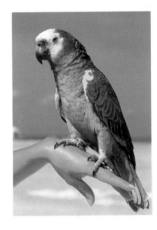

Parrots and cats are among the many pets that can cause an allergic reaction. For asthma sufferers especially, the only realistic solution is to avoid having a pet in your home.

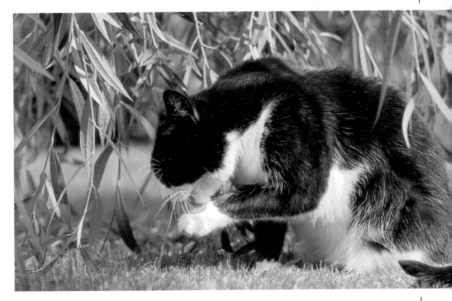

Irritants and allergies at work

Even if your home is allergen-free, you may be exposed to allergens at work. It is estimated that about one in 330 of the working population may be affected by occupational asthma, but the figure is probably greater.

The most common form of occupational allergy is allergic inflammation of the skin, known as contact dermatitis. Occupational asthma—symptoms triggered by your work—accounts for 2 percent of all adult asthma and is the second most common form of workplace allergy. Some workers also suffer from a runny nose (allergic rhinitis) and red itchy eyes (conjunctivitis).

Occupational asthma and allergies are an important cause of work-related illness, but they are not widely known. Some people are reluctant to complain to their employer for fear of losing their job, but ironically, every year thousands have to give up their work because of occupational asthma.

Indoor irritants

Anybody who comes into contact with particles small enough to be inhaled is at risk. There is a long list of chemicals that can trigger allergies, but two of the worst offenders are di-isocyanate—particularly toluene di-isocyanate, used in spray painting and work involving urethane varnishes or foams—and colophony fumes, given off during soldering. In hospitals, technicians have become allergic to the chemicals used in the processing of X rays.

Office equipment and furniture can emit toxic chemicals, and sealed windows—a feature of many offices—mean that these hazardous substances do not readily disperse.

Not all irritants at work are chemicals. Bakers may be allergic to flour dust, laboratory workers to proteins found in animal urine, and workers in food-processing plants to salmon, crabs, prawns, or shrimps.

It is not only factory and farm workers who are exposed to substances that could trigger an allergic response. Modern offices can also be hazardous places. Printers and photocopiers give off toxic gases and particles, and the equipment is often not in a room by itself. In addition, rooms are usually poorly ventilated. Items of furniture such as carpets and office seating can "out-gas," in other words, give off gases. Carpets, for instance, can exude a cocktail of harmful gases including formaldehyde, toluene, and benzene.

If you spend much of your time working around the home doing renovation projects, you could easily come into contact with a number of noxious chemicals. Formaldehyde causes dryness and irritation of the throat and can affect the eyes and air passages. It is an allergen that few people know about but it is everywhere—in chipboard, plywood, paper, cosmetics, photographs, foam rubber, and leather luggage. Even when you can no longer smell it, it can give off gases for 20 years.

Latex gloves

Workers in hospitals and dentist offices need to wear latex gloves to protect them from infections, including HIV and

IS WORK MAKING YOU SICK?

You can be fairly sure that work is causing your problems if:
- *Your symptoms start soon after you have started a new job or soon after your job conditions have changed.*
- *The symptoms get better on the weekend and during a vacation.*

There are two types of occupational asthma. The most common type is latent occupational asthma, which develops when you have been working at your job for some time; this explains why new workers or apprentices in some industries experience fewer and less severe symptoms than their more experienced colleagues.

The second type is when you have symptoms of chest tightness, wheeziness, shortness of breath, and a dry cough almost immediately. This is usually because of the high concentrations of allergens in the air.

Some people have a late-phase reaction—their symptoms occur not only during work but also for several hours afterward as well. Their wheeziness or rash may last over the weekend, which may obscure the true source of the allergens.

hepatitis. The gloves are dusted with a fine starch to lubricate them and this starch bonds to the latex proteins in the gloves and carries them into the air.

These particles can cause asthma and dermatitis in one in 10 of those who wear latex gloves or who regularly come into contact with latex. If someone who is allergic to latex is operated on by a surgeon wearing latex gloves and latex enters their bloodstream, they can go into anaphylactic shock. If you know you have an allergy of this type, make sure you tell the surgeon at your initial consultation.

If you work in an environment such as a hospital, where the air is full of latex proteins and you develop an allergy, you may have to leave your job. Just avoiding latex will probably not be enough. A study of hospital staff in Finland showed that 3 percent were allergic to latex. A survey in a Canadian latex glove factory revealed that 3.7 percent of workers had asthma caused by latex.

Sick building syndrome

In a modern office building, allergens of all kinds are recycled through air ventilation systems. Perfumes, dry-cleaning fluids, printers' ink, and tobacco smoke can circulate around an office, causing untold misery to an allergic individual.

In addition, mold spores grow in the air ducts and water tanks and are circulated around the office. Dust mites also live in the furniture. Some scientists now believe a leading cause of sick building syndrome is gases given off by molds and fungi that thrive in the damp conditions found in air-conditioning systems. Molds such as aspergillus and mildew produce gases such as benzene that can cause allergic reactions in the immune system. Damp winters and humid summers are ideal conditions for mold growth, and air-conditioning systems are particularly fertile breeding grounds.

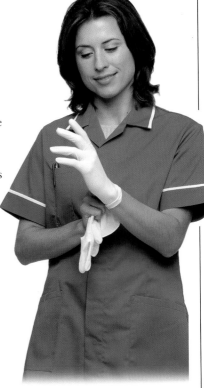

The latex gloves worn by health workers for protection can cause an allergic reaction. There are alternatives, but they are expensive.

Drugs and additives

*I*nhaling cigarette smoke, both actively and passively, can make you susceptible to asthma attacks, and ingesting a variety of substances ranging from food colorings to drugs can prompt an allergic reaction, taking forms ranging from a rash or wheeziness to anaphylactic shock in the most severe cases.

The evidence linking smoking with several serious diseases is now overwhelming. If you suffer from asthma, smoking can only make it worse.

Smoking

Almost everyone today knows that smoking is bad for you. And yet between 15 and 20 percent of people with asthma still indulge in the habit, even though it makes them more wheezy. Pregnant women who smoke increase the risk of the baby being asthmatic and having other respiratory illnesses.

Tobacco smoke contains some 4,000 chemicals, present either as gases or tiny particles. Nicotine stimulates the central nervous system, increases heart rate, raises blood pressure, and is highly addictive. Tar, the sticky brown substance that gathers at the filter tip of a cigarette, sticks to the lungs and is gradually absorbed. It contains a cocktail of noxious substances, including formaldehyde, arsenic, cyanide, benzene, toluene, and carbon monoxide, all of which interfere with red blood cells, making them carry less oxygen around the body.

Passive smoking

You don't have to smoke to inhale fumes. Every time you walk into a bar you will get a blast of tobacco and if your asthma is severe you should avoid such places. Other people's smoking habits can make your life a misery and if you live or work with a smoker there is little or no escape from smoke-related risks.

There are many studies linking asthma and cigarette smoke. In one survey 8 out of 10 people said a smoky atmosphere made their asthma worse. Research shows that 28 percent of pregnant women who work are exposed to smoke at work.

Passive smoking doubles the chance of a child developing asthma. Children of smokers are more likely to have episodes of wheezing and need time off from school than those with nonsmoking parents. It is generally worse when the mother smokes because many children spend more time with their mother than their father.

Chronic coughs and phlegm are more common among children of parents who smoke. Children of parents who smoke inhale nicotine in amounts roughly equivalent to smoking 60–150 cigarettes each year.

Food additives and flavorings

Processed foods contain an enormous number of additives to color, flavor, and preserve them. There are about 3,500 additives, though some are natural. They are difficult to avoid and it has been estimated that we eat around 10 lb (4.5 kg) of additives a year, with people in some countries, such as the United States, consuming far more.

Some doctors believe that high doses of these additives can lead to children becoming hyperactive, accident prone, irritable, easily distracted, restless, and unpredictable. Research at child health institutes has shown that artificial colorings and preservatives are at the top of the list for causing problems associated with attention deficit disorder, or hyperactivity, and other researchers have found that some artificial colorings may interfere with digestion.

Many people who have allergies would like to place the blame on food additives, but in reality not many additives actually cause an allergic response. However, a few do and some countries, particularly in Scandinavia, ban their use. Additives that are not approved in the European Community do not have an E attached to their number.

Some doctors believe that chemicals used to coat food, such as insecticides, fungicides, and herbicides, also trigger asthma. Ethylene gas, used to ripen bananas, and paraffin wax, used to give a sheen to peppers, cucumbers, and apples, may also set off an asthmatic reaction.

Monosodium glutamate, a flavor enhancer commonly used in Chinese food and as a meat tenderizer, has been shown to bring on asthma symptoms and a variety of other reactions, of which migraines are the best known.

Drug allergies

You may experience side effects of the drugs you have to take, but serious allergic reactions to medication are rare. It is not always easy to distinguish an allergic reaction from a recognized side effect. If you have a bad reaction to a medicine it is important to tell your doctor so that it goes down in your medical records. You may forget your adverse reaction, but your body's immune system has a good memory that will last for years. You are more likely to develop an allergy to a drug you take occasionally and to one that is injected than to one you swallow regularly.

Chief culprits

• Aspirin and other nonsteroidal anti-inflammatory drugs (NSAIDs) can bring on an asthma attack in around 2–4 percent of asthmatics, particularly middle-aged women. Symptoms of such an aspirin-induced attack may include a rash, flushing, and a runny nose as well as a narrowing of the airways.

These everyday drugs, along with the food additives tartrazine and benzoic acid, hamper the production of substances called prostaglandins. Prostaglandins are found all over the body and are involved in pain perception and so an effective painkiller will act on them to stop their production.

But prostaglandins also affect the airways, some relaxing them and others constricting them. In an asthmatic person, aspirin and NSAIDs can upset the delicate airways that are already inflamed, triggering an attack.

• Antibiotics (amoxicillin and trimethoprim are the main offenders) can produce a nasty rash. It is unlikely that you will be allergic to all antibiotics, so your doctor will make a note of the ones that cause a reaction and ensure that you are given a different one next time. If you develop a rash shortly after starting a course of antibiotics, consult your doctor and pharmacist for advice. Do not continue the course unless you are advised to do so. Antibiotics can cause anaphylactic shock, though this is rare. If you do have this allergic reaction, you should avoid all aspirin products as well.

• Antitetanus injections can cause anaphylactic shock.

Home solutions

For many people a house is not a home if it does not have central heating, wall-to-wall carpets, comfortable furniture, and heavy curtains. But if you or any member of your family has asthma, then you may not be spending your money wisely. Research shows that it would be better to strip the floorboards, put up blinds, and buy leather chairs.

Keep dust mites out of your bedding with microporous covers. Washing bed linen at high temperatures is another recommended measure.

The best way to fight asthma and allergies is not to become sensitized in the first place. A study of 67 children in the United Kingdom and the United States showed that early exposure to the house dust mite sensitized the children, and their sensitivity was in direct relation to the level of mites found in their homes. The message was clear: bring up your children in homes free of carpets, with the windows open and the heating down low, and they will grow up healthy and asthma-free.

So what can you do to keep your home allergen-free? Research points to the fact that dust mites are killed by freezing, by temperatures over 131°F (55°C), strong sunlight, dry cleaning, and some chemical sprays. You should vacuum or dust surfaces with a damp cloth—dry dusting dislodges clouds of allergens into the air.

Bedding

There is a hundredfold reduction in exposure to dust mites if mattresses, duvets, and pillows are covered with special microporous covers that let water through but stop mites from getting in. These covers are much better than the old plastic ones that are slippery, impermeable, and have a tendency to grow mold on the inside.

Every week, covers should be wiped down and allowed to dry because mites gather on top. Sheets, pillow cases, and duvet covers should be washed once a week at temperatures of 140°F (60°C) or higher. If your freezer is big enough, put bed linen in a plastic bag in the freezer overnight, defrost it, and wash it at a high temperature. Lower temperatures will not kill the mites.

Furnishings

Choose a bed with a plain wooden or metal frame rather than a divan base, and have a plain headboard, not an upholstered one. If you have bunk beds for your children, the child with asthma should sleep in the top bunk.

Avoid upholstered furniture in the bedroom and if you are buying furniture for your home, choose chairs covered in leather or nonfabric material. If you have upholstered furniture, vacuum it once a week. Blinds are better than curtains, but if you have curtains, wash them every two or three months.

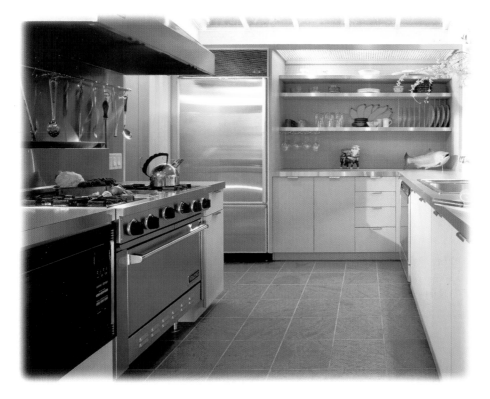

Tiled flooring, wipe-clean surfaces, and the absence of soft furnishings contribute to an allergen-free environment.

Flooring

Carpets are wonderfully warm underfoot, but they provide a haven for house dust mites. You can cut the number of dust mites dramatically by removing the carpet and replacing it with cork tiles, linoleum, or vinyl flooring. Stripped, sealed floorboards look wonderful anywhere in the home and they can be enlivened by short-pile rugs.

But some scientists now believe that many people have gone too far, ripping up their carpets and reducing their bedrooms to bare, prisonlike cells. While admitting that carpets are dwelling places for dust mites, many doctors are now saying that ventilation is just as important. If possible, sleep with your windows open—the fresh air will help keep your chest decongested and kill off dust mites. ▶

VACUUM CLEANERS

Every day thousands of people scrub and vacuum their homes from top to bottom to make their house mite-proof, but their efforts may be in vain. The dust mite sticks stubbornly to its chosen habitat and no matter how thorough you are with your vacuuming, the mites cling on. Even if you do remove some of them, the remainder breed rapidly and will make up their losses within a week.

Vacuuming may not remove mites, but it is better to vacuum than not, if only to remove the droppings and dead mites. Invest in a vacuum cleaner designed for the job—there are plenty to choose from—and vacuum when the person with asthma is not around. Vacuuming stirs dust into the air for about half an hour.

Ordinary vacuum cleaners often have bags that are porous, and the mite droppings that escape the bag are blown out via the exhaust. Some models of vacuum cleaner have tougher bags and exhaust filters. These catch the mite droppings and seal them inside the vacuum cleaner.

Home solutions

Pets and toys

Despite the fact that pets, particularly cats, harbor a mass of allergens, most people enjoy snuggling up to them. But even if you avoid touching or stroking an animal you can still have an allergic response since the allergen spreads quickly through the house.

One solution, and probably the best, is not to have an animal in the house. However, if you can't part with your pet—and this could be a very difficult decision for many families—air your home, make sure the pet doesn't wander into the bedroom, and encourage it to spend more time outdoors.

Some doctors recommend you simply regularly wash pets and their bedding.

If you can take it away from your child, once a week put a soft toy in a plastic bag and leave it in the freezer overnight. Low temperatures kill dust mites and their eggs.

This greatly reduces the number of allergens they carry, although anyone who has ever tried to bath a cat once, let alone regularly, will know that this may not be a realistic solution.

For children, soft toys may be even harder to part with than pets, but they do attract mites. Freeze overnight in a plastic bag to kill the mites, and if the toy is washable, wash it at 140°F (60°C).

Cleaners and chemicals

Acaracides are chemicals that kill dust mites and ticks. You should spray your carpets and furnishings at least twice a year—it is important to vacuum thoroughly afterward. This will remove not only the dead mites but also their asthma-triggering droppings.

The chemicals used are tannic acid, crotamiton and benzyl benzoate. But these chemicals themselves can cause skin irritation. Some doctors maintain that acaricides have little impact on dust mite levels.

Air filters and ionizers

The air is full of tiny dust particles that have a positive or negative charge. Ionizers work by changing the positively charged particles in the air to negative, which removes them from the air. Ionizers are cheap but they do not make a significant dent in the number of allergens in the air. Similarly, although electrostatic air cleaners can clean a smoky bar, they don't make much of an impact on allergens.

High-efficiency particle air filters do reduce the level of airborne allergens, but they do not control the "clouds" of

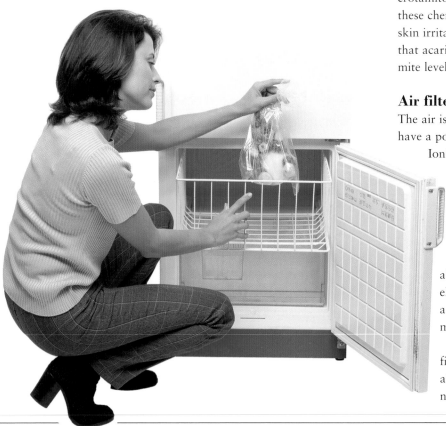

allergen created by movement. The ideal place for these filters is in low-traffic areas of your home, such as the bedroom.

Clothing

There is no evidence that wearing cotton is better than wool when it comes to lessening the risk of an asthma attack, although cotton blankets are better than wool ones. But whatever you wear, remember that clothes may also be full of dust mites and you should wash them regularly at 140°F (60°C).

If you have sensitive skin and suffer from skin allergies, you may find that wool irritates you and makes your eczema worse. This is not only because wool can be scratchy but also because of the natural lanolin it contains.

Condoms

Some people are allergic to condoms, which may give them (or their partner) itchy or sore genitals. It is not usually the rubber that causes the problems but chemical additives that are used in the spermicidal agents.

Most manufacturers of condoms offer low-allergy alternatives, which are made from nonallergenic materials and have a water-based lubricant that does not contain spermicide.

Humidity

Air the bedrooms and living rooms every day to cut down on the humidity. During the pollen season, do this at night, when there is less pollen in the air. Dry clothes outside or in a tumble drier—not over a radiator—and fit extractor fans in the bathroom and kitchen.

A damp house not only provides a haven for mites, it also encourages mold growth. Make sure your house is well

Find out more	
Allergens in the home	40
Outdoor solutions	54

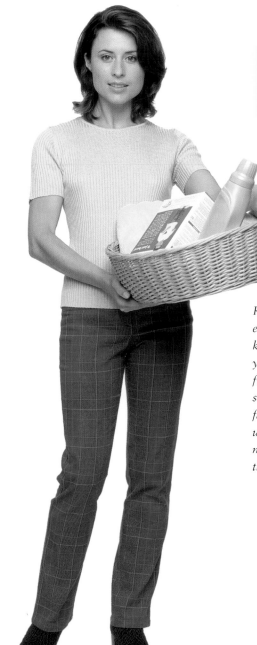

Regular washing is essential in the battle to keep the dust mites out of your clothes. If you suffer from eczema and find some soap powders and fabric softeners make it worse, double-rinsing may help to eliminate this problem.

damp proofed—houses built before 1920 often are not. A diligent rountine is necessary to combat dampness. Mop up condensation on the window sills, use air conditioners and dehumidifiers, and wash shower curtains regularly.

Outdoor pollution

People often associate air pollution with billowing smoke from factories and thick smog. But automobile exhaust is also a significant source. And even pollutants that we can't see may aggravate breathing problems.

Most pollutants are caused by burning fuels, such as gasoline, coal, and diesel. Although air pollution from industrial smoke and sulfur dioxide has lessened, other types of pollution have increased. The number of cars on the roads has risen, and exhaust fumes have increased in some countries by almost three-quarters.

Main outdoor pollutants

• Nitrogen dioxide (NO_2) is found in vehicle exhaust and is on the increase. However, NO_2 exposure is greatest in a home with a gas stove and gas heaters.

• Carbon monoxide is another gas emitted by cars. It reduces the amount of oxygen in the blood and high levels cause headaches and drowsiness.

• Nitrogen oxides (nitrogen dioxide and nitric oxide gases) cause acid rain and smog. They irritate the lungs and aggravate asthma.

• Ground-level ozone is produced on sunny days and is a by-product of exhaust fumes and factory pollution. Large amounts of ozone can damage the lungs and immune system. Ironically, levels of ozone are thinning high up in the upper

IRRITANTS IF YOU WORK OUTDOORS

SUBSTANCE	OCCUPATION
ANIMAL PRODUCTS, especially urine	Laboratory workers, animal breeders, veterinary practitioners, farmers
GRAIN MITES	Farmers
INSECT PRODUCTS	Workers rearing silk worms, maggots, butterflies, bees
MOLD SPORES	Farmers, construction workers, renovators working on old buildings
PESTICIDES	Farmers, agricultural workers
VEGETABLE DUST	Coffee, tea, tobacco, and soybean workers
WOOD DUST	Carpenters, wood turners
WOOD PRESERVATIVES (formaldehyde, lindane, pentachlorophenol)	Anyone handling wood

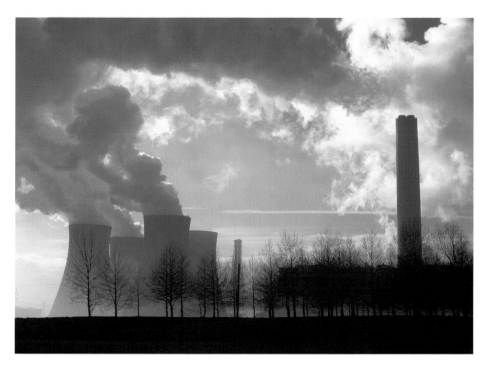

Power plants, cars, trucks, and heavy industry are among the main contributors to atmospheric pollution.

atmosphere where ozone protects us from the harmful effects of ultraviolet light.

• Sulfur dioxide (SO_2) is produced when coal is burned. Its main source is power plants. It makes breathing problems worse by tightening the airways. In cities, levels of SO_2 are boosted by vehicle exhaust emissions.

• Acid air is caused when gases such as nitrogen oxides and sulfur dioxide react with water vapor. Not much is known about its effects.

• Particulates are sooty specks of dirt whipped up by the wind, or produced by burning coal or diesel fuel. They are what makes traffic smell dirty. Heavy goods vehicles and diesel cars pump out around one quarter of the particulates in the air, though in cities this figures can be far higher. Very small particulates can pass deep into the lungs and aggravate breathing problems.

• Volatile organic compounds (VOCs) are smog-forming gases, such as polyaromatic hydrocarbons and benzene. Benzene, which is known to cause cancer, escapes from exhausts and gasoline pumps when you are filling up the car.

Effects of pollution

Studies have shown that hospital admissions for asthma are higher when levels of pollution are high. Other studies have shown that high volumes of traffic lead to respiratory difficulties in children.

But researchers now think that other triggers, such as the house dust mite or pollen, may affect asthma sufferers more than air pollution. And there is no evidence that air pollution causes asthma. Studies in Eastern Europe show low levels of asthma despite heavy air pollution. Cities such as Los Angeles and Mexico City also have heavy pollution but low rates of asthma.

Outdoor solutions

Pollution may not be the cause of asthma, but it can make it worse. Unless you cover yourself from head to foot there is little way of avoiding outdoor pollutants completely. However, there are commonsense steps you can take.

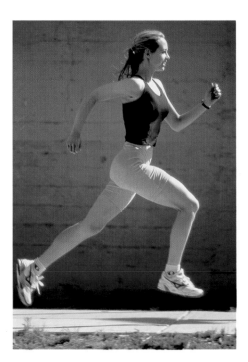

Exercising in moderation can be beneficial and strengthen the lungs. But it is better not to go out jogging in cold, dry weather. Avoid areas with heavy traffic.

• When pollution is really high, there will be air-quality warnings on the television or radio. Tune in and avoid going out when pollution is very high.

• Don't jog in polluted areas and if you live in a city and cycle to work, wear a mask.

• If you are experiencing asthma or allergies at work, get in touch with your union if you belong to one.

• If you or any of your family suffer from asthma, try to avoid living near a busy road or a factory that spews out pollutants into the air.

Pollen counts

Most pollen is released from the grass in the morning, rises into the air in the heat of the day, and can be blown for many miles, right into cities. When the air cools in the evening the "pollen cloud" comes down and the count falls.

The pollen count ranges from 30 to 400. It is measured by an instrument that sucks in air and calculates the number of pollen grains per cubic meter of air averaged over the previous 24 hours. The point at which hay fever symptoms are triggered depends on the type of pollen that is present. A count of 50 is enough to trigger symptoms in most hay fever sufferers.

On rainy or windy days the pollen count tends to be low; but dry, slightly breezy days are ideal conditions for the pollen to lift off the plant. If you don't know what pollen count triggers your symptoms, keep a diary of the pollen

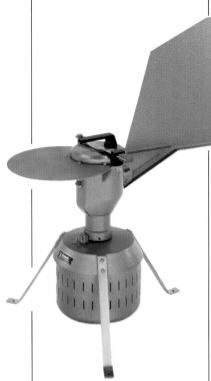

A pollen count meter provides scientists with the data to calculate the average pollen count—vital information for the hay fever sufferer. The instrument pictured here is a seven-day recording volumetric spore trap.

SUNGLASSES

Researchers have found that making shields with paper or clear plastic around the sides of glasses can stop pollen from entering the eyes and is much more effective than wearing unadapted glasses. Many people with hay fever are also sensitive to strong sunlight, and sunglasses are a welcome relief.

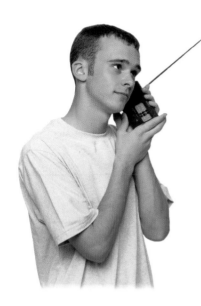

During the pollen season, radio stations give details of the pollen count, often with the weather report. They will also broadcast air-quality warnings.

count and the severity of your symptoms and look at it afterward to match up symptoms and pollen count.

How to avoid pollen

One of the best ways of tackling hay fever is to avoid pollen. The following list gives some suggestions as to the measures you can take during the pollen season:
• Avoid areas of long grass.
• Wear sunglasses when you go out to reduce the number of pollen grains reaching your eyes.
• Drive with your car windows closed. If possible, choose a car with a pollen ventilation system.
• As the pollen count rises in the afternoon, close the windows.
• Sleep with the bedroom windows closed when the pollen count is high.
• Wash your hair and clothes after spending a day in the garden or countryside.
• Get your partner or a friend to mow the lawn and stay away while they do so.

• A stroll on a summer's day might sound romantic, but the pollen count is at its highest at that time.
• Take summer breaks on the coast where sea breezes keep the pollen inland.
• Avoid picnics or camping vacations during the high-pollen season.

Quitting smoking

The chemicals in cigarette smoke irritate the lungs, which in someone with asthma are already inflamed. If you have asthma, smoking is about the most dangerous thing you can do and the best thing to do is stop.

Many smokers fear that if they quit they will put on weight. Some people do indeed gain weight, but usually only a few pounds, which are lost in a matter of months. Smoking reduces the appetite so when you give up cigarettes, food tastes better and you eat more. Moreover, many smokers enjoy a cigarette after a meal. When you quit smoking that may be replaced by a second helping or a dessert. If you are hungry, snack on fresh fruit and vegetables.

If you feel you need hypnotherapy, acupuncture, nicotine patches or chewing gum to help you, by all means use them, but sometimes all they do is put off the day when you throw away the cigarettes, ashtray and lighter. You will have a tough couple of weeks and you will need the support and tolerance of friends and family, but it will be worth the effort.

You may experience withdrawal symptoms, such as irritability and sleeping problems. Be proud that you have given up smoking, take it one day at a time, and congratulate yourself at the end of the day. Don't be tempted to have "just one" cigarette. It will probably lead to another ... and another.

Cycling is generally a healthy activity. But in heavy traffic, wear a mask to protect your lungs from the pollution.

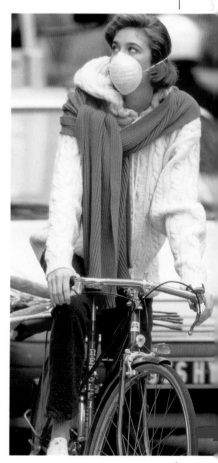

Stress

*I*t *is only recently that doctors have turned their attention to stress. They now recognize that it affects our health in all sorts of ways. Some people react to stress by having a headache; others find that their digestion is upset and they may develop irritable bowel syndrome.*

Research has shown that stress, both major stresses, such as bereavement or the breakdown of a marriage, and minor, or micro, stresses, have a marked biochemical and hormonal effect on the body. Stress may greatly reduce our ability to cope with life's demands. Conversely, the hormones released when you are under stress give you the push and incentive to meet deadlines and targets, and are the fuel of ambition. Sometimes this stress buzz is what is attractive about a job —most newspaper journalists and financial traders feel at their most productive when they are under intense pressure.

But stress can also bring on an asthma attack and make many allergies, particularly eczema, considerably worse. It cannot cause them, but it can trigger them. Many parents with an asthmatic child have to resign themselves to birthday parties bringing on an attack because of the combination of excitement and exercise.

Asthma and allergies are certainly not all in the mind, but the mind has a powerful impact on them. This may explain why a number of complementary therapies, which aim to restore a healthy mind–body relationship, have had success in treating asthma.

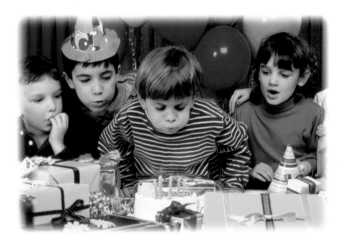

The overexcitement at a children's party is an all-too-familiar cause of the onset of an asthma attack.

Boosting the immune system

The mechanism whereby stress affects your body and can damage your health is complex. The mind and body communicate through pathways, the study of which is so important that it now has its own name—psychoneuroimmunology (PNI). The immune response is controlled by the brain through the autonomic nervous system, which regulates activities such as heartbeat, sweating, flushing, and hair erection and is largely outside your control, and the endocrine system, which controls your hormones.

While the immune cells send out shock messages to the brain that something has invaded the body, it is the central nervous system that responds and constricts the airways, or causes the skin to erupt into lumps, or sends the body into a state of anaphylactic shock. It also increases the number of protective white blood cells the body produces at this time of crisis. When you are under temporary stress the brain releases hormones that boost the immune system's ability to fight off invaders. During chronic, or long-term, stress, the body is unable to maintain these increased hormone levels and the number of natural killer cells decreases, leaving you more open to infection. The stress hormones cortisol and epinephrine flood into the blood stream, increasing the heart rate and raising the blood pressure. Your rate of breathing will increase, you may perspire more, and your digestion may be upset. Long-term stress results in high blood pressure, anxiety, irritability, aches and pains, breathlessness, palpitations, and sometimes depression. The raised cortisol levels may weaken your immune system and you may develop skin rashes, food intolerances, and eczema.

Power of the mind

Scientists are only just beginning to understand the power of the mind over the body. If you are the sort of person in whom emotion and stress could trigger an asthma attack, the mere suggestion that you are inhaling an allergen is enough to make you wheeze.

Studies have shown that when people with asthma were told that they were breathing mist from an aerosol containing substances to which they were allergic, they were likely to have an attack, even if the aerosol contained only a harmless salt solution. If they were told they were inhaling medication that would make their breathing better, their breathing would improve, even if it was only the same salt solution.

Exercise

People are constantly being told to exercise, and for most of them, regular exercise can only improve their health. But for asthmatics, exercise can cause breathing problems. This is called exercise-induced asthma.

Research has shown that in 8 out of 10 children with asthma, running for five minutes reduces by 15 percent the peak expiratory flow rate, that is, the maximum speed at which they breathe out. Children who do not suffer from asthma might be a bit out of breath after running but their peak expiratory flow rate remains the same.

Children with asthma may cough and wheeze a few minutes after they start exercising, while teenagers and adults may cough after they come off the football field or tennis court. It is ironic that many athletes have exercise-induced asthma.

For parents, having an asthmatic child poses a constant dilemma. Should you let your child run around with other children, like any healthy child, and risk an attack, or keep her at home and never let her run free? Such a life might be psychologically as well as physically damaging. But many parents do this and the pale, thin, wrapped-up child with shoulders hunched through spending too many hours in front of a television set or a computer is a sign of the times.

Exercise may bring on wheeziness and coughing, but it tends not to cause the acute attacks that allergens such as pollen and the house dust mite trigger. So it is important to let your child exercise, even if it has to be done gently. Exercise strengthens muscles and the heart, improves the circulation, lowers blood pressure, and improves agility.

Find out more

Immune system	26
Extreme allergic reactions	30
Relaxation	102

Competitive sports combine extreme tension with vigorous exercise and can provoke respiratory problems.

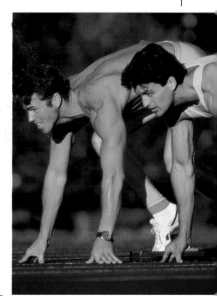

Stress solutions

O ne of the best ways to tackle stress is to relax. Everywhere we turn, magazine articles, radio and television shows, and our friends and family urge us to take it easy. But relaxation, for many people, can be as difficult as giving up smoking.

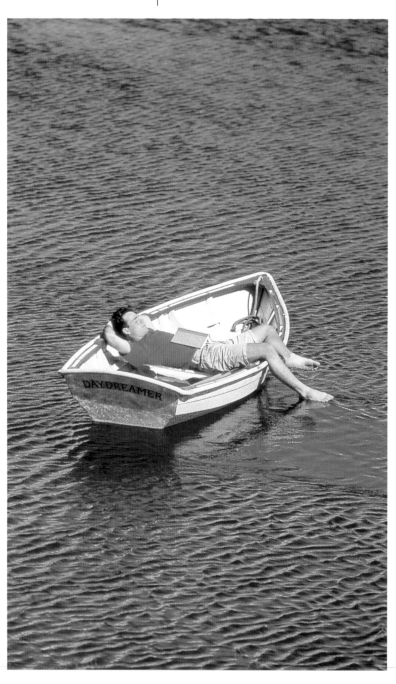

Many of us have been brought up to believe that we are only worthwhile if we are achieving something—that is, doing something. If we are not doing something then we are being idle and idleness equals laziness and unproductivity.

Relaxing and switching off, whether you are sitting quietly reading a book or doing something more active like playing golf or football, can be difficult. You may be stretched out on the sofa in front of the television, but you may be in a state of tension, particularly if what you're watching is gripping.

True relaxation comes from taking time out to do nothing but relax. When you are truly relaxing, changes happen in your body that can help asthma—muscles relax, epinephrine levels subside, blood pressure lowers, breathing becomes slow and deep, brain waves alter, and you become calm and focused.

Try to set some time aside for yourself every day just to relax. This may be easier some days than others, but don't give up. There are plenty of ways to help yourself—you can meditate, practice t'ai chi or yoga, master autogenics or self-hypnosis—or just learn simple breathing techniques. When relaxation becomes part and parcel of your life you will have better control over your asthma, and allergies, such as eczema, may recede.

Many people today have to learn how to relax. Don't feel guilty about taking time off from your busy routine—it can be a valuable part of controlling your asthma.

And remember, don't keep your feelings to yourself. Just telling someone, whether it's a colleague, friend, partner, or counselor, about the things that are making you anxious can bring enormous relief. One study has suggested that 6 out of 10 people who had experienced serious asthma attacks were in denial. A healthy emotional attitude can go a long way toward combating stress.

Exercise precautions

• Don't go for a cross-country run on a cold, dry day or during the height of the pollen season.
• Always do warm-up exercises before you start exercising.
• Take medication before exercising—two puffs from a reliever inhaler should be enough. Take medication rather than cutting back on exercise.

IS THERE AN ASTHMATIC PERSONALITY?

There is some evidence that certain characteristics may single you out as being at risk and make you more likely to develop asthma than other people. Various studies have suggested that asthmatics are irritable, angry, obsessive, and prone to depression. They bottle things up and hide their feelings when they are tense. Some doctors say tension is reflected in the lungs and air passages, and there have been cases where releasing repressed emotions and fears has alleviated asthma.

It is difficult to know what comes first—the asthma or the personality traits. Having a condition that makes you wheezy and breathless is depressing, and if you are living with a condition which means you have to clean the house from top to bottom to banish house dust mites or patches of mold, then it is all too easy to become obsessive about your asthma.

Nevertheless, a number of studies show that anxious and depressed sufferers are more likely to be wheezy, wake breathless or with a tight chest,

and have attacks of breathlessness when resting or after activity.

Some children can deliberately bring on an attack by hyperventilating or coughing unnecessarily, in order to win sympathy, manipulate their parents, or avoid school. There is little doubt that a few people find that their eczema or allergy can win sympathy and attention. This is known as secondary gain.

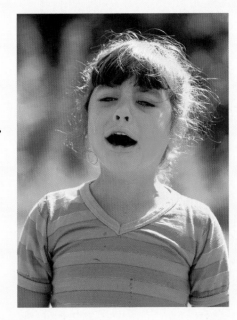

Tests for asthma and allergies

ome asthma symptoms are present in other conditions, such as coronary heart disease, bronchitis, or emphysema. So breathing tests are used to pinpoint asthma and eliminate other diseases from the diagnosis. The two main devices for testing lung function are the peak flow meter and the spirometer.

Peak flow meter

If you have asthma your airways become narrowed so the air will not flow freely. It is impossible to measure the diameter of the air passages, but this can be estimated by finding out the speed at which air is expelled from the lungs.

The peak flow meter, or peak expiratory flow meter, is a small instrument that measures the maximum rate at which you breathe out. You take a huge breath, inflating your lungs as far as you can, hold it for a couple of seconds, then force it out into the device as fast as possible. As you breathe out the speed of the air quickly reaches its peak, then drops off. The instrument registers the fastest speed.

These are inexpensive instruments and your family doctor will have one. You can also buy one for yourself and use it to monitor your peak flow two or three times a day. The peak flow meter is invaluable for warning you that your condition may be deteriorating. Using this device regularly could save your life.

The volume of air expelled by a healthy lung is between 88 and 132 gallons (400 and 600 liters) per minute. In asthma rates of between 44 and 88 galllons (200 and 400 liters) are common and in severe attacks it could drop to 22 gallons (100 liters) a minute or lower.

Spirometer

A more sophisticated piece of equipment, used in hospitals and chest clinics, is the spirometer. It measures the amount of air expelled in one second, or forced expiratory volume in one second (FEV1), and "forced vital capacity," that is, the volume of air expelled in one breath.

If your lungs are in good shape you will take about four seconds to breathe out fully and most of the air—about 70 percent—will be expelled in the first second. If you have asthma, only half or even less of your breath will be exhaled in the first second.

The spirometer gives more detailed information, but it cannot give you the regular daily readings that you will get from a peak flow meter.

Bronchial reversibility test

The bronchial reversibility test measures your breathing before and after using a bronchodilator. If your peak flow improves by 15 percent or more after a puff of the bronchodilator, you may have asthma.

The Vegatest machine measures the electromagnetic field you produce when you are exposed to a certain substance. Some allergists find this useful in identifying the cause of an allergic reaction.

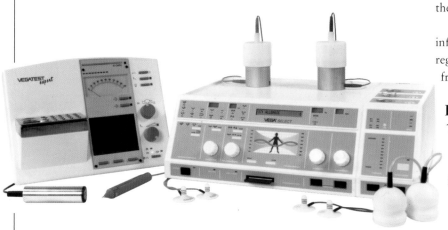

ALLERGY TESTS

● *Skin prick test*

This is the most common test used to pinpoint allergies. You can be tested for up to 25 allergens at any one time.

Small amounts of the suspected allergen are pricked into the skin of the back or forearm with a tiny prong about $1/25$ in (1 mm) long. You won't be injected with anything and it won't hurt. If you are allergic to a substance you will develop a wheal, a small bump that may be itchy and red around the perimeter. The doctor will measure the wheal after about 15 minutes and anything bigger than $1/12$ in (3 mm) will be regarded as a positive result.

This test is a good indication of the substances to which you may be allergic, but it is not foolproof. Some allergens, such as pollen, dust and fungi, "perform" better than foods, which are unreliable.

Similar tests include the "intradermal infection" test, which produces a wheal and is not common; and the patch test, where the suspect substance is placed on a small patch of lint and stuck on the skin for between 48 and 72 hours.

● *Radioallergosorbent test (RAST)*

This is a blood test that measures the number of special allergy antibodies (IgE) your immune system has produced to a particular substance, such as pollen, the house dust mite, or a food protein. A small quantity of your blood is taken from a vein and sent to a laboratory for testing. Here a drop of your blood serum will be applied to a sample of the allergen.

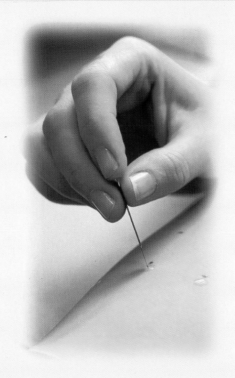

The test uses a technique whereby a radioactive marker attaches itself to the IgE cells and the total quantity of radioactivity is measured at the end of the test.

Measuring the quantity of IgE in the blood after it has been applied to a particular substance and comparing it with the quantity of IgE in your blood stream shows how allergic you are to that substance.

This test is often used in conjunction with the skin prick test as well as in cases when a skin prick test is not suitable. For instance, you may have extensive eczema or you may be so severely allergic to something that there is a risk that you might have an anaphylactic reaction.

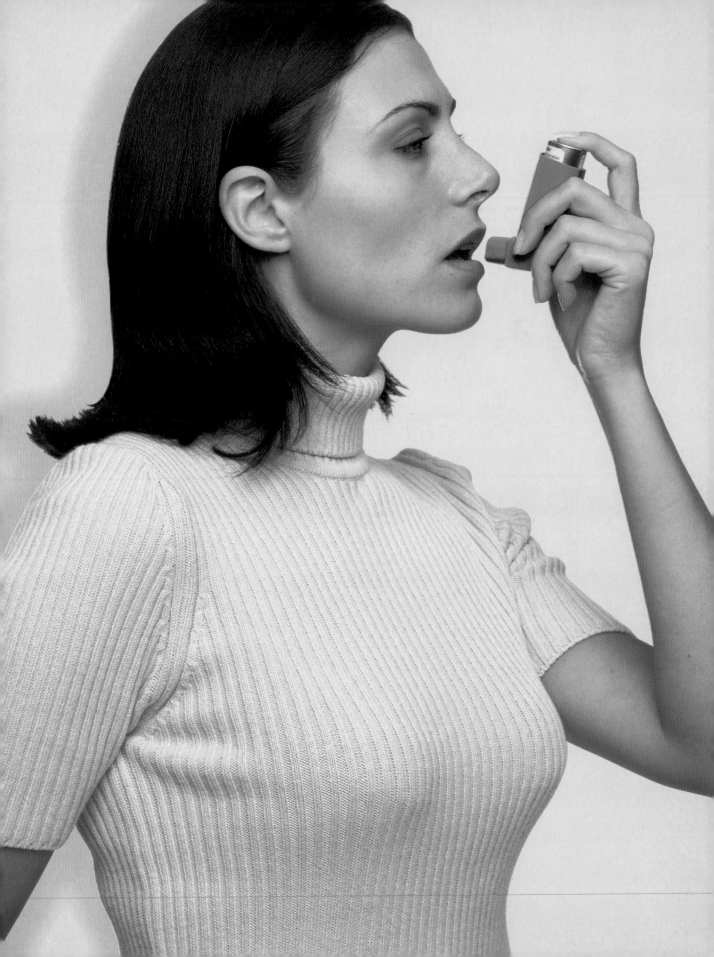

3
CONVENTIONAL
THERAPIES

Today's treatments for asthma are effective and easy to administer yourself. You may be worried about the side effects of drugs that you are taking every day. For example, you may fear that bronchodilators can cause nausea, hyperactivity, and hyperventilation and that taking steroids may be harmful in the long term. You may have heard that these drugs might actually make your asthma and allergies worse. But asthma is a serious condition and sometimes powerful drugs are needed to treat it.

As yet there is no drug that can cure your asthma or make your allergies disappear. What drugs can do is relieve your symptoms so that you can lead as normal a life as possible.

Drugs for asthma

I*f you have asthma your medication will be divided into three groups—preventers, relievers, and emergency drugs—taken via a bewildering array of delivery devices.*

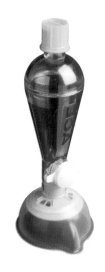

A spacer is a plastic container that when fitted to an inhaler is filled with a fine mist of medication. A mouthpiece at one end allows you to breathe in normally, which means it is easier to use than an inhaler alone.

Relievers relax the muscles in the airways so that they open out and you get more air into your lungs. These drugs are called bronchodilators and may be beta-agonists such as ventolin (which enhance sympathetic activity) or anticholinergics such as atrovent (which reduce sympathetic activity). You usually inhale them. They may give you immediate relief if you are having an attack, so you should always carry your inhaler around with you. Preventers tackle the underlying inflammation, so calming the airways, and are steroids.

Preventers

These are anti-inflammatory drugs, or steroids that prevent your airways from becoming inflamed. They can be inhaled, taken as tablets or, in severe cases, injected. Inhaled steroids are the most common.

Corticosteroids—steroids for short—prevent the airways from becoming inflamed. They only work if taken regularly. Corticosteroids were developed from the natural body hormone cortisol, which is produced by the adrenal gland. The steroids used to help asthma are extremely effective in stopping the inflammation and swelling of the airways and the accumulation of mucus in the lungs—they damp down the allergic reaction.

While a steroid is a powerful drug, it is safe because you breathe in only a minute amount and, in the prescribed dose, it goes directly to where it is needed—the lungs. For preventers to be effective, they must be taken regularly, twice a day. For someone

who suffers from asthma and allergies this may seem wonderful, but steroids have to be taken with care because if you take more than the prescribed dose—and in some cases, even if you take the prescribed dose for any length of time—there can be side effects.

Steroids can be inhaled, swallowed in tablet form to relieve an acute attack or to control severe asthma, or injected for a severe attack. Injections are always given by a doctor or nurse.

Inhaled steroids are breathed in using an inhaler (puffer), a spacer, a dry-powder inhaler, or occasionally a nebulizer. The most widely used drugs are budesonide, beclomethasone, and fluticasone.

Unlike bronchodilators, used as relievers, inhaled steroids must be used every day, even when you are feeling fine—over time they will gradually reduce the inflammation. If you stop taking your preventer medicine when you are feeling well, your symptoms will gradually return. It is important that your dosage is "stepped down" or reduced when your asthma has improved. The maintenance dose should be the minimum necessary to keep your symptoms at bay.

There are few serious side effects from a regular standard dose, but you may feel a bit hoarse and you may develop candida, a yeastlike fungal infection in the mouth that may cause a sore throat.

The most widely used steroid tablet is prednisolone. This is prescribed when inhalers don't work for you. Your doctor may advise a short course—a week or two—of these tablets if you have had a sudden severe attack, or you may be given a longer course to give you control over severe chronic asthma.

Relievers

These drugs give instant relief because they act on the muscles of the airways, relaxing and widening them. Bronchodilating drugs are usually inhaled, but can be taken as tablets or syrup.

Short-acting drugs work very quickly and relieve symptoms for three to six hours. They are taken by inhaler and should be taken as required. Long-acting drugs relieve symptoms for up to 12 hours and are often taken at night. They can be inhaled or taken as tablets and are not recommended for children. Such drugs are good if you have moderate to severe asthma, particularly if your symptoms keep you awake at night, and for people with exercise-induced asthma.

Beta2-agonists

The most popular bronchodilators are a group of drugs known as short-acting beta2-adrenoreceptor agonists, usually called beta2-agonists, of which salbutamol and terbutaline are the best known. Adrenoreceptors are the places at which the "fight or flight" hormone, epinephrine, acts. Epinephrine makes you breathe faster, relaxing your airways so that you draw in more oxygen. An agonist is a drug that works on the receptor cells and mimics the real thing. In other words, it acts like epinephrine. When you take a puff from your bronchodilator, your lungs will "think" you have naturally released epinephrine and your airways will relax.

You should use your reliever only when you need it, that is, when you feel wheezy, out of breath, or have a cough. The effects should usually last for about four hours. ▶

ARE YOU USING YOUR INHALER PROPERLY?

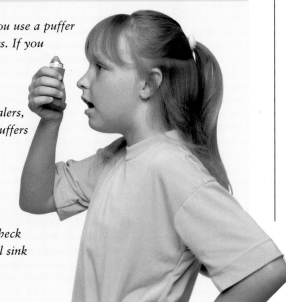

Puffers look simple, but are quite complicated to use properly. If you use a puffer incorrectly the medicine won't get to where it is needed—your lungs. If you don't synchronize pressing your inhaler and breathing in, most of the medication will end up in your mouth and throat, rather than in your airways.

In one study, 100 people were carefully trained to use their inhalers, but when they were tested later, only a handful always used their puffers correctly. The most common faults were:

• *Not shaking the puffer before use*

• *Not pausing or exhaling slowly*

• *Not waiting one to three minutes before each new puff*

• *Not coordinating puffing and inhaling*

• *With a nonmetered puffer, not knowing when it was empty. To check how low your inhaler is, float it in bowl of water. If it is full, it will sink —an empty one will float.*

CHAPTER THREE

Drugs for asthma

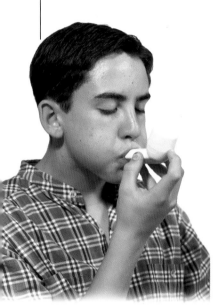

A dry-powder inhaler is convenient to carry, easy to use, and can provide fast relief from the symptoms of asthma.

If you find the relief the medication gives does not last this long, it is a sign that your asthma is not under proper control and you need to see a doctor. Longer-acting beta2-agonists are now available, and can be useful for nocturnal asthma sufferers.

Xanthines

Your doctor may prescribe a drug containing theophylline which belongs to a group of chemicals called xanthines, found in many plants, and in tea and coffee. A cup of strong coffee may prevent a mild asthma attack.

Theophylline drugs are taken in tablet form and work by relaxing the muscles around the bronchi and unblocking the airways. They are slowly released into your gut over 12 hours. In severe cases aminophylline, another xanthine, can be given as an infusion.

Anticholinergic agents

These drugs keep the air passages open by reducing the tendency of the airways to close under the influence of acetylcholine,

which has the opposite effect from epinephrine and tends to constrict them. By reducing the effect of acetylcholine, these drugs relax your airways for 8 to 12 hours. They are particularly useful for treating chronic asthma when anti-inflammatory medication and beta-agonists have not worked.

Mast cell stabilizers

These bronchodilating drugs work by making the mast cells in the lining of the lungs more stable, so preventing them from releasing the allergic chemicals, histamine and leukotrienes. With fewer of these chemicals in the body the allergic reaction will be weaker. The drugs are used as an alternative to beta2-agonists and are particularly good if you have exercise-induced asthma. Children tend to respond better to these drugs than adults.

New inhalers

Over the next few years, puffers will be replaced with new inhaler devices that do not contain chlorofluorocarbons (CFCs). The CFCs do not harm you, but they do

DELIVERY DEVICES

• A simple metered dose inhaler, often called an MDI or puffer. Bronchodilators are pale or sky blue, while relievers are brown or orange.
• A breath-activated large volume spacer for those who have difficulty using a puffer. Wash it out once a week since the drug may stick to the sides due to a build up of static electricity.
• Other breath-activated devices include the Turbohaler, Diskhaler, and Autohaler.

• Dry-powder inhalers (Spinhaler, Rotahaler).
• A nebulizer that creates a mist of asthma medication, which you inhale through a mask or mouthpiece. It delivers a much larger dose of the drug than a puffer and is used when you are experiencing a serious asthma attack. Most family doctors, all ambulances, and hospitals should have them and if you or your child has severe attacks you may have to have one at home.

ASTHMA DRUGS

PREVENTERS	**Inhaled steroids:** Methylprednisolone, prednisolone, betamethasone, dextamethasone **Oral steroids:** prednisolone, beclomethasone, budesonide, dipropionate, fluticasone propionate, hydrocortisone, cortisone, prednisone, triamcinolone, flunisolide
MAST CELL STABILIZERS	Sodium cromoglycate, sodium nedocromil
RELIEVERS	**Beta2-agonists:** *Short-acting:* salbutamol, terbutaline, fenoterol, pirbuterol, reproterol, rimiterol, tulobuterol *Long acting:* salmeterol, eformoterol, bambuterol **Xanthines:** Aminophylline, choline theophyllinate, theophylline **Anticholinergics:** Ipratropium bromide, oxitropium bromide

Find out more

Respiratory system	18
Drugs for hay fever	68
Side effects	76

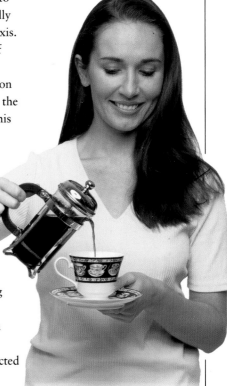

Coffee can help relieve asthma. Since it speeds the heart rate, it acts in much the same way as epinephrine.

damage the the earth's ozone layer. If you are being supplied with a new model, check with your doctor, nurse, or pharmacist that you know how it works.

Desensitization techniques

A large range of conventional therapies is used to tackle asthma and allergies. Treatments for hay fever and other allergies are detailed on pages 68–73.

If drug treatments and diet therapy do not offer sufficient relief from your asthma, you may be offered immunotherapy. There are several techniques but all involve regularly taking doses of the substance to which you are allergic, or that triggers your asthma, so that in the end—and the treatment may take several years—you develop a tolerance to the substance.

In hyposensitization or incremental desensitization, increasing amounts of the allergen are injected under the skin until your sensitivity to it is reduced. This is reserved for individuals with allergies to specific substances. It has to be carefully monitored due to the risk of anaphylaxis. A few children have died as a result of this treatment.

More widely used are desensitization or neutralization techniques, of which the Miller technique is the best known. This involves using a dose that just fails to cause a reaction and then giving that dose repeatedly. Practitioners of this technique claim that it is totally safe because of the small amounts used but you have to be committed to the treatment, which involves injecting yourself daily or every other day.

Enzyme-potentiated desensitization (EPD) is effective in the treatment of asthma and hay fever. Patients are injected four times a year with a cocktail of minute doses of allergens.

Treatments for hay fever

Many people are wary of taking drugs, particularly for something that seems as mild as hay fever. But apart from taking away the pleasure of a warm summer's day, hay fever can be debilitating, making sufferers feel tired and run down and unable to do anything without constant sneezing and coughing.

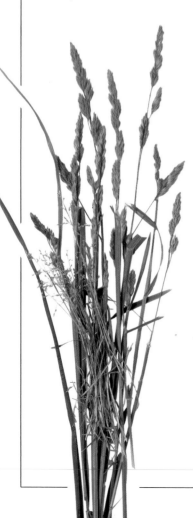

Pollens from grasses are the most common and widespread triggers of hay fever. Avoid them as much as possible during the pollen season.

There are three main types of medication for hay fever: antiallergy drugs, antihistamines, and corticosteroids. Like all allergies, hay fever can also be treated by desensitization techniques.

Antihistamines

These drugs are the most popular way of controlling hay fever symptoms. They come as tablets, capsules, or a liquid, and you can also buy eye drops containing antihistamines. A nasal spray is now available, and others are being developed.

They work by blocking histamine, one of the chemicals released by your body in an allergic reaction. Histamine causes red, itchy swollen eyes and an overproduction of mucus, and it makes you wheeze because it narrows your air passages. Antihistamines are good at reducing most of the symptoms of hay fever within an hour or two, but they do not clear a blocked nose.

Older types of antihistamine may cause drowsiness. This is because the histamine molecule sometimes interferes with other body chemicals, including epinephrine. You may become tired because epinephrine is being blocked. The newer antihistamines have been modified to cause little, if any, sleepiness.

Antiallergy drugs

These are sometimes called mast cell stabilizers and they nip the allergic reaction in the bud by damping down the activity of the mast cells. This medication can control "hay fever" eyes and a runny nose, as well as being good for asthma. It is usually taken as eye drops or a nasal spray. Itchy, red, and inflamed eyes can be soothed with sodium cromoglycate eye drops. A new drug, lodoxamide, acts in a similar way.

Steroids

These work in much the same way as drugs for asthma by preventing inflammation. Used in a nasal spray they reduce inflammation in the lining of the nose and so prevent a runny nose, a blocked nose, and sneezing. They can also help prevent red and itchy eyes.

If you suffer from severe hay fever, doctors recommend that you start taking steroids every day just before the start of the hay fever season and continue taking them until the end. Corticosteroids are available as tablets and you can also have a steroid injection.

Decongestants

Most decongestants belong to a group of drugs called sympathomimetics. They work by contracting the blood vessels in the nose, which reduces congestion and makes it easier for you to breathe. They usually come as nasal sprays, with the result that only a tiny amount of the drug enters your bloodstream. However, if you overuse the spray—or take decongestant tablets—you may have a few side effects, such as an increased heart rate and trembling.

Desensitization techniques

The aim of immunotherapy is to desensitize you to the substances that trigger your allergy. The technique was introduced at the beginning of the 20th century and works roughly in the same way as a vaccine. You are given a minute amount of an offending substance and over a period of time you gradually build up a resistance to it, so that after several treatments you are not allergic to it any more.

There are three main types of desensitization technique—incremental desensitization, neutralization, and enzyme-potentiated desensitization (EPD).

Incremental desensitization

Also known as hyposensitization, incremental desensitization gradually builds up your tolerance to a particular allergen by using progressively higher concentrations until a level is reached that will give you protection but will no longer cause any allergic symptoms.

The technique is used for hay fever and other seasonal allergies and anaphylaxis caused by insect stings. It can also be used for people who suffer specific animal sensitivities. Extracts made from insect venom can give 98 percent protection from wasp stings and 80 percent from bee stings. However, incremental desensitization is not suitable for skin allergies or allergic rhinitis and it has a low success rate with food allergies and intolerances. It is vital that this is monitored by your doctor.

Neutralization

In this treatment low doses of an allergen are administered daily or every other day by an injection just under the skin or by drops placed under the tongue. It is popular in the US and Australia but, apart from a few of clinics in the United Kingdom, the technique is not common anywhere else. The Miller technique, named after an American, Dr. Joe Miller, is exactly the same as neutralization.

Enzyme-potentiated desensitization (EPD)

This is a technique in which an enzyme called beta-glucuronidase is added to a weak solution of the allergens that trigger your attacks. The solution varies according to how severe your allergy is. There are two standard forms of treatment: it can be injected into the skin of the forearm or administered by the cup method.

In the cup method, a small area of the forearm or thigh is scratched to remove the waterproof layer of skin and the fluid is held over the scratch for 24 hours by means of a small plastic cup, fixed firmly to the skin. Treatment continues until you are no longer allergic to whatever it is that triggers your attacks.

Beta-glucuronidase is contained in every cell of the body, and EPD practitioners—all of whom are medically qualified—say this makes the body accept the desensitization fluid as a "friend" and create new cells that do not react to the allergen. After months of reprograming the immune system finally becomes "tolerant" to the allergen.

Unlike neutralization techniques, EPD is administered every few months. Initial doses tend to be every two or three months for one or two years. You may then have an injection once every four months and, following about the eighth injection, you may need any further injections only once or twice a year.

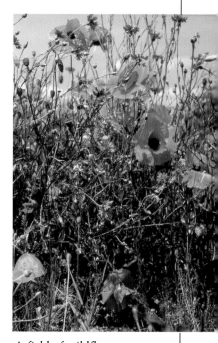

A field of wildflowers may be the source of a number of airborne allergens. It is a good idea to take your hay fever medication with you if you are going out for a walk in the country.

Treatments for skin allergies

There is no conventional cure for skin allergies. However, they can be brought under control and over time they may disappear by themselves. You can often make skin allergies clear up simply by avoiding whatever irritates the skin, whether harsh detergents, perfumed soap, or wearing wool or latex.

You can choose from a number of products that help with skin allergies. They include shampoos and skin creams to moisturize and soothe the skin and tablets to reduce irritation.

A number of treatments improve dry skin, making it less itchy and reducing inflammation, so there are lots of things you can do to make eczema easier to live with. Your doctor will offer advice about how to avoid allergies, but you may also be given a steroid cream, preparations containing coal tar, antihistamines, and antibiotics. If the treatment you have been given fails to work for you, don't use more and more of it. Go back to your doctor and ask to be given a different treatment or try complementary therapy.

Topical steroids

"Topical" means that the steroid or corticosteroid drug is applied to the skin rather than taken by mouth. It is the most popular form of treatment for eczema and comes in varying strengths—ranging from mild to potent— depending on how bad your eczema is and what part of your body it affects. Mild hydrocortisone cream should be available from

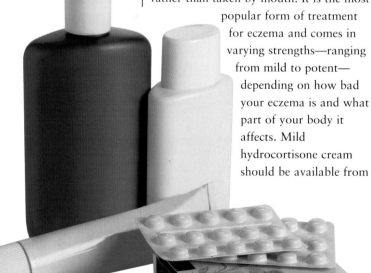

your pharmacist without a prescription, but if the condition persists you should consult your doctor. Topical steroids alleviate the symptoms, reducing itching, redness, and inflammation and allowing the skin to heal.

Emollients

There is a host of emollients on the market to soothe your skin. Emollients are a mixture of oils, fats, and water and come as creams, lotions, ointments, and bath oils to help restore the oil and moisture content of your skin.

Most people with eczema have dry skin, so a moisturizing bath oil can help. The bath water should be warm—not too hot or too cold—and the cream should be used immediately afterward.

Other skin creams

The most popular of these is coal tar, which comes as an ointment, cream, paste, or solution. It is good at thinning thick rough patches and may be enough to keep your eczema at bay. Tar is found in a number of preparations for eczema, but it is smelly and can stain clothing.

Other preparations include salicylic acid, which can smooth thick, scaly skin; zinc and calamine creams; and potassium permanganate dressings or baths.

Antibiotics

Eczema is not infectious, but because the skin cracks, is inflamed, and sometimes bleeds, you are open to infection from the germs that live on your skin. This infection is normally mild and can be kept under control by antibiotics.

If your eczema is severe, your doctor may also prescribe steroids, which are either taken by mouth or injected. The steroid most often used is prednisolone, used for asthma. It is sometimes prescribed when you are going through a stressful time in your life—such as exams —when a flare-up could be damaging to your career.

If you have atopic eczema you may have sore patches on your scalp, your hairline, and the back of your neck. Medicated shampoos may help. Many of these contain coal tar or an antiseptic. Give a shampoo a three-month trial.

Evening primrose oil

Gammalinoleic acid (GLA), or evening primrose oil, may ease your skin irritation. It is a natural oil from the seeds of the evening primrose plant and because it is oily it makes your skin smoother and less itchy. It is suitable for adults and children over the age of one, but it is best to ask your doctor's advice before you start taking it, particularly if you have epilepsy. If you do not notice an improvement after three months, there is no point in continuing with it.

Light therapy

If you have severe eczema or it fails to respond to topical steroids, your doctor may suggest light therapy, or PUVA treatment, which stands for "psoralen plus ultraviolet A." You will be asked to take a psoralen tablet and two hours later sit under a light, a bit like a sunlamp, which radiates a special kind of light. This type of treatment is used for both eczema and psoriasis.

Cyclosporin

The powerful drug Cyclosporin subdues the immune system and suppresses the allergic reaction. It is used in transplant patients to prevent the body from rejecting the new organ. However, though it is a lifesaver, it has serious side effects. For this reason, it is used only for adults with the most severe form of atopic eczema, and always under the supervision of a skin specialist.

Treatment with ultraviolet light and anti-irritant medication can be effective against eczema.

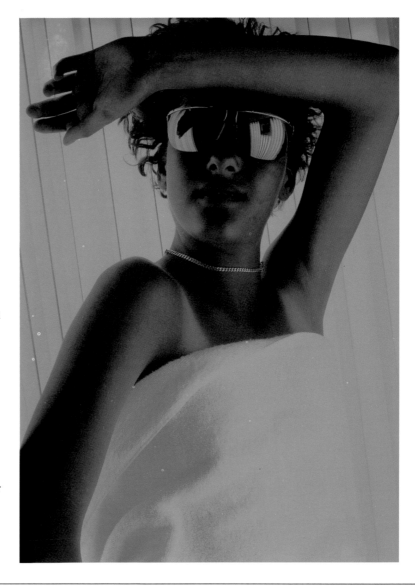

Treating food allergy and intolerance

True food allergies, in which the body's immune system reacts inappropriately to a harmless substance, are rare. However, you may be intolerant of, or sensitive to, a number of foods.

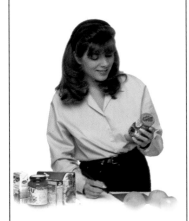

Even apparently harmless products can contain ingredients to which you are allergic, so you have to study all labels carefully.

It is estimated that only 1 percent of adults, usually men, and 5 percent of children have food allergies. In contrast, food intolerances are common and can lead to irritable bowel syndrome, eczema, and other conditions such as migraines, asthma, and rhinitis.

There is no drug therapy to treat food allergies. The only hope of a "cure" is to try neutralization or EPD techniques (see p. 69). However, the most effective way of reducing symptoms associated with food intolerances is to avoid those foods that disagree with you. The best way to find out which foods you cannot tolerate is an exclusion diet. Consult your doctor, then try the elimination diet suggested opposite.

To find out which foods upset you may require three to four months of food testing and repeated unpleasant reactions when "banned" foods are reintroduced. It sounds simple enough, but it is hard work giving up foods you may enjoy and which are part of your everyday life. There is no short cut. Although a number of tests have been promoted as quick ways of making a food intolerance diagnosis, studies have shown that none is reliable.

There is no scientific evidence that hair analysis or cytotoxic testing (in which a blood sample is taken and the white blood cells are mixed with food extracts) are accurate ways of assessing whether you are intolerant to certain foods. With a Vega machine, you hold one electrode and your toe or finger is touched with a second while different foods are introduced into the circuit. However, there is no proof that this can pinpoint your food intolerances and it could even do harm, since if you follow the "advice" obtained, you may become malnourished.

GLUTEN-FREE DIET

If your gut is especially sensitive to gluten, you may suffer from celiac disease, which can result in damage to the lining of the colon. If you think you have a gluten allergy your doctor may give you a simple blood test to identify cells known as antiendomyseal antibodies. If you have this antibody the chances are you have celiac disease.

The next stage is an intestinal biopsy, carried out by a gastroenterologist, in which a minute amount of the small intestine lining is snipped away via an endoscope, a fibre-optic tube that is passed down your throat and into your intestine. It's a quick and easy outpatient procedure and sounds more gruesome than it is.

Once diagnosed, there is no cure for celiac disease.

A life-long gluten-free diet is the best treatment. This is restrictive because you must avoid bread, rolls, pasta, buns, cakes, crispbread, and anything containing flour products, such as sausages.

It's not just the obvious foods you have to avoid. Ingredients such as tomato paste and stock cubes may also contain gluten, so read the label carefully and check whether the product contains wheat starch, rye, barley, or oats.

Supermarkets are beginning to sell gluten-free foods, and they are widely available from health food outlets, pharmacies, and specialist suppliers. If you want to bake your own bread buy gluten-free flour, or you could try rice, potato, or maize flour.

ELIMINATION DIET

WEEKS 1 & 2

Have a slow build-up to your diet: it's too much of a shock to the body to start the diet suddenly. For two weeks cut down on tea and coffee, then cut them out. Cut out fried food, fatty foods, alcohol, and red meat and anything you feel makes your symptoms worse. Limit consumption of butter, cheese, and milk.

If you're lucky, this may be enough to alleviate your symptoms. If not, start the full two-week diet. See your doctor before you do. Do not try this if you are frail, pregnant, or have a serious health problem. Keep a food diary and make a note of the foods that upset you.

DAY 1: Eat normally

Day 2: Fast, drinking only water. This is a good way of flushing out the toxins in your body. If you just can't take it or feel unwell, eat a banana. Take it easy—don't drive or do anything physically taxing.

DAY 3: Start following the short-term exclusion diet. For two weeks eat only the foods listed in the "Foods allowed" column below and none of the foods listed in the "Foods not allowed" column.

FOODS NOT ALLOWED	FOODS ALLOWED
MEAT Beef, sausages, hamburgers, meat products	**MEAT** All other meats and poultry
FISH Fish in batter or breadcrumbs	**FISH** White/fatty fish canned in brine/oils
VEGETABLES Potatoes, onions, sweetcorn, canned vegetables in sauce	**VEGETABLES** All other vegetables fresh/frozen/canned, salads, legumes, sweet potatoes
FRUIT Citrus fruits (oranges, lemons, grapefruit, limes)	**FRUIT** All other fruits fresh/canned
CEREALS Wheat, rye, oats, barley, corn	**CEREALS** Rice, arrowroot, tapioca, sago, buckwheat, soyflour, millet, rice cakes
DAIRY PRODUCTS Cow's milk, butter, most margarines, sheep/goat's milk and products, yogurt, cheese, and eggs	**DAIRY PRODUCTS** Soymilk, milk-free margarine, tofu, soya-yogurt
DRINKS Tea, coffee, alcohol, citrus fruit juice, artificial fruit drinks, tap water	**DRINKS** Herbal teas, noncitrus pure fruit juices, blackcurrant fruit drink, mineral water
MISCELLANEOUS Yeast, gravy mixes, salad dressings, mayonnaise, blended oils, corn oils, vinegar, nuts, chocolate	**MISCELLANEOUS** Salt, herbs, spices, honey, syrup, oils—olive, sunflower, safflower and soybean, dried fruit, seeds, carob

This diet should be followed strictly for two weeks. Try not to smoke. Foods should then be reintroduced in the following order at the rate of one every two days:

Tap water, potatoes, milk (12 fl oz/330 ml), yeast (3 brewer's yeast tablets or 2 teaspoons fresh yeast), tea, rye (rye crispbread or rye bread), beef, butter, *onions, eggs, oats, coffee, chocolate (try milk-free chocolate or cocoa), citrus fruits, corn, cow's cheese, wheat (test white pasta, flour, and bread; if you can tolerate yeast, try a wheat breakfast cereal or whole-wheat or granary bread), nuts, barley, vinegar.*

Managing your asthma

*I*t is important that you control your asthma, rather than *allowing* it to control you. Of course, it can be irritating to take medication and to think daily about activities and situations that could trigger an attack, but you must always be aware that uncontrolled asthma is dangerous.

It would be wonderful if everything to which you were allergic disappeared overnight, but even if you scrubbed your home from top to bottom and banned animals, you would still be surrounded by allergens. Once you have been diagnosed as having asthma, it's up to you to take responsibility for it. The best way to do this is to be alert to your symptoms and to check your peak expiratory flow (PEF) with a meter. Your doctor may help work out a self-management plan for controlling your asthma.

If you are managing your asthma well, you should live a normal, healthy life. You should sleep well at night, exercise normally, and need to use your medication only occasionally. If you combine this lifestyle with complementary therapies that suit you, you will be in control of allergies.

Peak flow readings

The peak flow meter is the best way to measure the condition of your lungs. Because peak flow tends to fall before you feel any symptoms, a reading also acts as an early warning system.

Strong and healthy lungs will expel between 88 and 132 gallons (400 and 600 liters) of air. In asthma sufferers, rates of between 44 and 88 gallons (200 and 400 liters) are common. During a severe attack this figure could fall even lower.

Peak flow readings vary from person to person so don't compare yours with anyone else's. Find out what your best reading is when you are in good health and symptom-free and use that as a benchmark. Base your management plan around your PEF readings. As a simple guideline, if your reading falls below 80 percent of your best reading, you may have to take more puffs on your bronchodilator.

With most plans there are two significant readings—80 percent and 60 percent of your best reading—and three zones: 80 to 100 percent, 60 to 80 percent, and below 60 percent.

• If your readings are regularly above 80 percent, your asthma is well controlled.

• If they drop between 80 and 60 percent, increase your medication.

• If the reading falls below 60 percent, you need to act quickly. Take a lot of your reliever drug (salbutamol or terbutaline sulfate)—up to 30 puffs. Take prednisolone tablets.

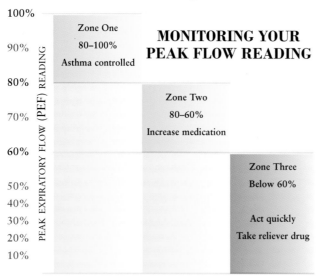

MONITORING YOUR PEAK FLOW READING

PEAK EXPIRATORY FLOW (PEF) READING

100% — 90% — 80% — 70% — 60% — 50% — 40% — 30% — 20% — 10%

Zone One
80–100%
Asthma controlled

Zone Two
80–60%
Increase medication

Zone Three
Below 60%

Act quickly
Take reliever drug

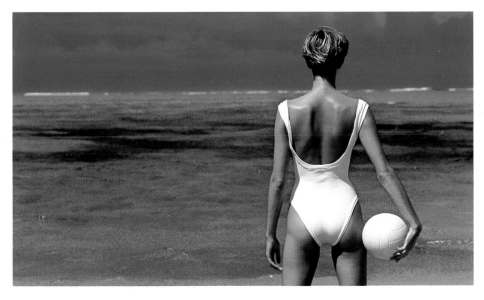

If you follow your asthma management program you should be able to enjoy life to the full. Take time to relax, breathe fresh air, and get some light exercise.

How to manage your medication

Many doctors now use "step" treatment plans, with each step showing you what treatment is needed to control your asthma. If the treatment recommended in one step is not controlling your asthma, then move on to the next one and so on.

Step 1

If you have few symptoms, you should only need to use your short-acting bronchodilator (salbutamol or terbutaline) once a day. If you are finding you are using it more than once a day you may have to go onto the next step.

Step 2

As well as your bronchodilator, you should regularly use preventive treatment—inhaled steroids—to reduce the inflammation in your lungs. The most common preventers are budesonide, beclomethasone, and fluticasone. Sodium cromoglycate and sodium nedocromil are alternatives.

Step 3

If your asthma is still not under control, you may have to take higher doses of preventers and your doctor may suggest you use a spacer.

Step 4

You may need to try a different type of short-acting reliever and a longer-acting reliever, as well as a high-dose preventer.

Step 5

As well as a short-acting reliever, a longer-acting reliever, and your high-dose preventer, you may need regular daily steroid tablets.

WARNING SIGNS

In addition to peak flow readings, there are other signs that your asthma is slipping out of control.
- *You need your reliever more often or the relief doesn't last as long as it used to*
- *You wake at night short of breath, coughing, and wheezing.*
- *You feel out of breath after your usual amount of exercise.*

   Don't increase your medication at the slightest dip in your readings. Some studies have shown that owning a peak flow meter leads to some improvement in management for people with acute asthma, but for others it neither reduces the frequency of attacks nor improves anxiety.

Side effects of medication

Few drugs are without side effects, but your doctor will probably feel that the risks associated with some medications are worth the benefits you will gain. If you are concerned about long-term use of some of these drugs, consult your doctor.

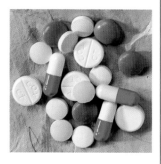

Drugs may be essential to control your condition—they may even save your life. But inevitably they have side effects, so it is important to monitor your medication carefully.

Bronchodilators

By relaxing the tiny tubes in the lungs, these drugs provide immediate relief during an attack when the tubes constrict, producing shortness of breath and wheezing. However, regular overuse of beta2-agonists can make your lungs worse, not better. Overuse interferes with the smooth lining of the airways, affecting the breakdown of magnesium, which prevents the airways from tightening. This makes them even more sensitive.

The more you use your bronchodilator, the greater the dosage you will need to achieve the same effect. These drugs can also have a rebound effect: if you stop taking your medication your asthma will be worse than before. Some doctors believe that overprescription of asthma drugs has contributed to the enormous rise in people suffering from asthma.

Researchers in New Zealand found that an asthma epidemic and a number of asthma deaths in the 1980s were caused by the high-dose bronchodilator fenoterol. They calculated that someone with severe asthma using fenoterol was 13 times more likely to die than someone using a low-dose reliever, because the drug stimulated the heart as well as the lungs.

Similarly, a study carried out in a number of medical schools in the United States showed that use of the drugs fenoterol and salbutamol, taken by a metered-dose inhaler, was linked with an increased risk of death and near death.

These risks are linked with very high doses. So it is important to use your bronchodilator only when you need it—doctors recommend that you don't use it more than once a day. It is vital always to follow your doctor's instructions.

SIDE EFFECTS OF BRONCHODILATORS

TYPE OF DRUG	BRAND NAME	SIDE EFFECTS
FAST-ACTING BRONCHODILATORS	Salbutamol, terbutaline, fenoterol, pirbuterol, albuterol	In higher than normal doses, these drugs will stimulate the heart; you may suffer from palpitations, a racing heartbeat, and abnormal heart rhythms.
LONG-ACTING BRONCHODILATORS	Salmeterol, theophylline, formoterol	It is dangerous to take too much theophylline, so if you are on this drug have a blood test periodically to check your level. Some other drugs, including antibiotics and antiulcer medication, increase the risks associated with theophylline.

Steroids

Inhaled steroids soothe the airways and, in the correct dose (below 800 mcg), should do you no harm, but use them sparingly. Used regularly, inhaled steroids can retard a child's growth and some studies have shown that in adults even low doses of inhaled steroids reduce bone formation.

Taken in larger than normal doses (1,500–2,000 mcg a day), steroids turn off the body's production of its own natural steroids in the adrenal gland. This increases the body's vulnerability to infection. In children taking steroids, illnesses such as the measles and chicken pox may be more serious.

In an emergency the adrenal glands normally release a surge of steroids to cope. This will not happen if you are taking high-dose steroids. It is vital to carry a steroid warning card at all times for at least two years after you have stopped taking steroids.

Overactivity of the adrenal glands and/or the taking of high-dose steroids over a period produces Cushing's syndrome. Typical symptoms are a red face, fat abdomen, buffalo hump on the back of the neck, muscle weakness, and high blood pressure. You may also gain weight. Your skin may become thinner and you may develop stretchmarks and acne. Women may become increasingly hairy. All these symptoms disappear when you stop taking the medication.

Inhaled steroids may make you hoarse and give you oral thrush. You can combat hoarseness by brushing your teeth after you've used your preventer, rinsing your mouth thoroughly. Eating yogurt with active cultures daily may ease thrush.

Xanthines

One study showed that aminophylline did nothing to speed recovery from an acute asthma attack or ease breathing. Side effects of the xanthines may include headache, nausea, and vomiting.

Drugs for hay fever

One of the antihistamines, terfenadine, which reduces symptoms without affecting alertness, has been linked to heart-related deaths. This drug is now available only by prescription. You should not take terfenadine if you have a heart or liver problem or if you take certain antibiotic or antifungal medications. If you do take it, do not drink grapefruit juice, which makes the blood absorb more of it.

Doctors believe that another new antihistamine, fexofenadine, is as effective as terfenadine without the side effects.

Decongestant sprays decrease blood flow to the nose and so reduce swelling. But if you use them too liberally, you risk damaging the lining of the nasal passages. Decongestant pills or low-dose steroid sprays do not cause this problem.

Find out more

Drugs for asthma 64
Treatments for hay fever 68

DRUGS FOR SKIN DISORDERS

Evening primrose oil may cause headaches, nausea, or indigestion. This can be overcome by taking it with food.

If you overuse topical steroids, your skin will become dry and thin, and tiny blood vessels close to the surface will become visible. The steroids will damage the tissue of the dermis, so stretchmarks may develop; these will be permanent. If you have dark skin, you may get temporarily reduced pigmentation in the area where you are applying it. You may also experience increased hair growth.

Antibiotic creams can cause irritation or allergic reaction. Itchiness is probably due to ingredients in the product and not the drug itself. However, if your skin becomes swollen, tell your doctor.

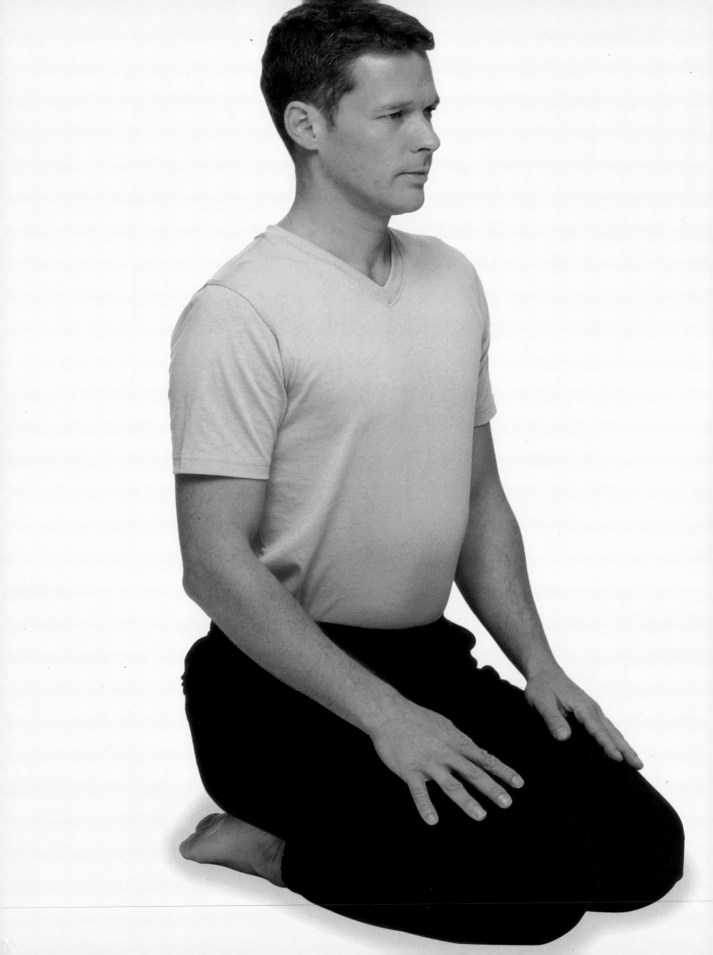

4

YOUR TREATMENT

OPTIONS

*S*ome allergic conditions, such as eczema,
respond well to complementary therapies
alone, but with asthma it is unwise to abandon
your conventional medication altogether, and no
reputable complementary therapist would advise
you to do so, even though the treatment may
enable you to cut down on the drugs you are
taking. Although it is understandable to be
worried about the effects of taking drugs every
day, remember that asthma medication is
effective and saves lives.

This chapter outlines a number of complementary
therapies, which may help relieve your condition.
Treatments range from self-administered
therapies, such as yoga and aromatherapy, to
practitioner-administered ones, such as
acupuncture, herbal medicine, and osteopathy.

Why complementary medicine?

Forty years ago complementary therapies were dismissed as "fringe medicine" and most people put their faith in doctors, who had time to talk to their patients. Now conventional medicine seems so rushed and increasing numbers of people are turning to complementary medicine.

Your doctor can supply you with any number of pills, creams, lotions, and inhalers to keep your symptoms at bay and most of them do what they say they'll do. Itchy skin settles, blocked airways relax, sneezing stops, and eyes clear. Sometimes this medication can save your life. So why are more and more people turning to complementary medicine and using it alongside—or even instead of—orthodox treatment? Is it really a good way of dealing with serious conditions like asthma and severe eczema?

Doctors may be able to scan and X ray every part of your body and even manipulate your genes, but some doctors have become removed and remote. Many people feel that their doctor is interested only in their lungs or their skin.

One of the attractions of complementary medicine is that the therapies are holistic—therapists treat the whole person, the mind and spirit as well as the body. They believe there is a close relationship between your body, your emotions, and your spirit or soul, and that your body's energy should flow freely among all three. Such practitioners believe you become ill when your energy is sluggish or blocked and they will work on your body to free up that energy and restore health.

An acupuncturist would call this energy *qi* or *chi* and tell you that it flows along an invisible network of pathways called meridians. A yoga teacher would say that energy passes through invisible holes in the body, called chakras.

While conventional medicine can cure killer diseases, it is not good at dealing with chronic conditions—ailments that go on and on because there is no drug to cure them. Asthma and most allergies fall into this category, along with many types of back pain, migraines, irritable bowel syndrome, and chronic fatigue.

Your doctor can keep symptoms at bay, but if you stop taking the medication, they may return, often worse than before. Also many of these ailments may have a psychological origin, caused by difficulties at work or at home, poor housing

The healthy functioning of the lungs is, of course, a vital part of the body's survival mechanism. When the tubes carrying air to the lungs become inflamed an asthma attack occurs.

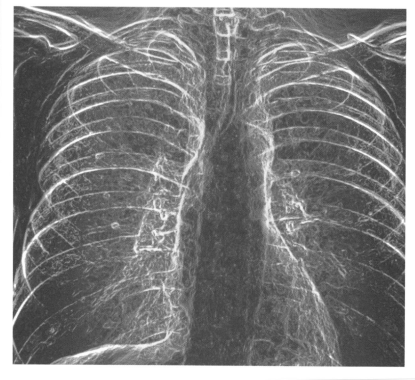

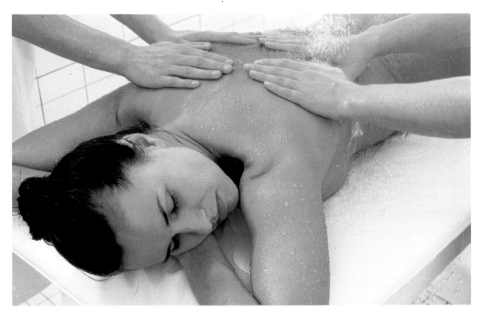

Find out more

Stress 56
Choosing a complementary practitioner 150

The therapeutic benefits of massage are now widely recognized. It reduces stress levels and induces relaxation, which may help clear up eczema or stave off an asthma attack.

conditions, and so on, and they derive much benefit from the holistic approach.

Complementary medicine can certainly help people with asthma and allergies. Some therapies help reduce stress and anxiety. Others may boost your energy levels by working along the meridians using fine needles or finger pressure, or you may drink an herbal tincture or take a homeopathic remedy.

With all of them you will be taking control and thus taking responsibility for your own health. Instead of being the patient taking medication from your doctor and hoping that the symptoms will go away so that you can get on with your life, you will become aware of your own needs, both physical and mental.

For many people, nonorthodox medicine offers hope and a way of living with whatever it is that afflicts them. It may even offer a cure. Equally important, it also builds self-confidence.

Some complementary therapies deal with chronic diseases extremely well and do so without harmful side effects.

Through complementary medicine you can learn how to harness your energy by relaxing, eating the right foods, breathing properly, and increasing your mental and spiritual well-being. It means looking at the causes of your illness in addition to the symptoms.

WARNING: PRACTITIONERS

You may have reached the end of the road with conventional medicine and feel that it can offer you nothing more. But be careful in your choice of complementary therapist. In some countries, anybody can practice complementary medicine, so it is important to consult a practitioner who is registered with an appropriate organization.

Apart from the fact that a poorly trained therapist could harm you both physically and psychologically, you may be put at risk because he or she fails to recognize a disease for which there is good orthodox treatment. Complementary medicine is harmful when it gets in the way of a proper diagnosis and effective treatment, so always visit your doctor before you visit a therapist. Be extremely wary of a practitioner who suggests you stop taking your medication.

Choosing a therapy

WHICH THERAPY IS RIGHT FOR YOU?	
BREATHING TECHNIQUES (pp. 86–89)	Breathing techniques are based on the belief that many people breathe poorly and don't use their lungs to their full capacity. This hyperventilation leads to stress, tiredness, tension, and a host of chronic conditions such as asthma. By learning how to breathe properly you can restore yourself to health.
YOGA (pp. 90–93)	Yoga is a spiritual and mental discipline that consists of a system of exercises designed to promote health and well-being. Through yoga the body is toned, the lungs are fully used, and the spine is kept supple, strengthening your vitality.
T'AI CHI/QIGONG (pp. 94–97)	T'ai chi is a series of gentle, graceful movements flowing into one pattern, or form. Qigong (pronounced "chee gung") is a related ancient Chinese system of exercises in posture, breathing, and mental discipline. Both are designed to promote health and well-being by restoring the flow of vital energy, or *qi*, around the body.
AUTOGENIC TRAINING, VISUALIZATION (pp. 98–99)	Autogenic training aims to bring about mental and physical well-being by auto-suggestive exercises that combat stress, improve creativity, bring about relaxation, and stimulate the body's self-healing mechanism. Visualization harnesses the power of the imagination to help fight illness, combat stress, and achieve potential.
MEDITATION (pp. 100–101)	Practiced regularly, meditation brings about a deep relaxed state that destresses you and can help stress-related conditions including asthma and allergies.
RELAXATION (pp. 102–103)	True relaxation requires concentration. Breathing becomes slower and deeper, blood absorbs more oxygen, and muscles relax fully.
AROMATHERAPY (pp.104–105)	Aromatherapy employs the essential oils of plants, each of which is believed to have different therapeutic qualities.
ACUPUNCTURE/ ACUPRESSURE (pp. 108–110)	Acupuncture has been practiced for 5,000 years. Through the insertion of fine needles at specific points it improves or unblocks *qi*, which flows around the body along invisible pathways, called meridians. Acupressure works on the same principle but finger pressure is used instead of needles.
SHIATSU (pp. 110–111)	Shiatsu is an ancient Oriental massage therapy using finger, palm, or foot pressure on various parts of the body. This increases vitality, releases tension, eases pain, and increases the ability of the body to heal itself.
HERBAL MEDICINE (pp. 112–119)	Herbal medicine, both Chinese and Western, uses plant remedies to treat disease. The aim is to build up the body so that it fights off illness and heals itself.

WHICH THERAPY IS RIGHT FOR YOU?

AYURVEDA (pp. 120–121)	Ayurveda is the traditional medical system of the Indian subcontinent. It aims to restore healthy balance through diet, massages, herbal remedies, and yoga.
HOMEOPATHY (pp. 122–123)	Homeopathy is based on the idea that "like cures like." A homeopath will treat you with tiny amounts of a substance that in healthy people causes the same symptoms.
OSTEOPATHY/ CHIROPRACTIC (pp. 124–127)	Although there are differences between them, these therapies are both methods of manipulating joints and muscles to correct musculoskeletal misalignments.
ALEXANDER TECHNIQUE (pp. 128–129)	Alexander technique treats the body through posture. Once you have achieved postural harmony and learn to use your body correctly, bodily functions such as breathing, circulation, and digestion improve.
NATUROPATHY/ NUTRITIONAL MEDICINE (pp. 130–135)	Naturopathy aims to enable the body to heal itself through fasting, diet, hydrotherapy, and exercise. Nutritional medicine is similar, and aims to restore health through diet and supplements.
HYDROTHERAPY (pp. 136–137)	Hydrotherapy is the use of mineral waters and thermal springs to restore health.
MASSAGE (pp. 138–141)	A massage relaxes muscles and improves blood flow by stimulating the lymphatic system. There are many different kinds, from the relaxing Swedish massage to vigorous Chinese massage, known as *tuina*, or deep Indian *marma* massage.
HEALING (pp. 142–143)	Healing is believed to work through spiritual or cosmic energy that flows through the hands of the healer and into your body, transforming disease and bringing about well-being. It is sometimes called laying on of hands.
REFLEXOLOGY (pp. 144–145)	Reflexology is based on the theory that the organs and all parts of the body are linked via channels that end in the feet or hands. A reflexologist will use gentle pressure on the feet to treat disease by unblocking these energy channels.
BIOFEEDBACK (pp. 146)	Biofeedback is a method of controlling biological functions by monitoring them with an instrument, which gives you feedback.
HYPNOTHERAPY (pp. 147)	Hypnotherapy brings about an altered state of consciousness through deep relaxation. Once you are totally relaxed, the therapist will make suggestions to free you from underlying stress and anxiety that may make your symptoms worse.

Self-administered therapies

The effects of disciplines such as meditation, t'ai chi, and qigong are profound, but they are not a quick fix nor will they instantly reduce symptoms. Many people say that practicing such techniques affects their whole lives, making them calmer and stronger, both physically and mentally.

If our lives are not filled with things to do from dawn to dusk we feel we are not fully functioning. Instead of facing up to our problems, we run around filling our lives with commitments and obligations, adding to our stress, and squeezing out any time for ourselves.

Stress is not all bad; if we didn't have the spur of stress, we would achieve little. But if we lead stressful lives we must learn how to cope with stress effectively. Unless we learn to relax and discharge stress, at the same time recharging our "energy" batteries, we will begin to show signs of chronic tension, such as ulcers, headaches, digestive disturbances, and allergies.

We may relax and the world may momentarily stop when we light up a cigarette or have a few drinks, but in the long term these quick fixes will not ease the stress that may be contributing to asthma or allergies and indeed may add to our tension. Real relaxation comes through a regular stilling of the mind, achieved through meditation, prayer, relaxation techniques, or calming exercises, such as t'ai chi. All these can easily be learned and incorporated into our lives. They give us a short space in the day when we can "sign off" from our daily pressures and hassles and allow ourselves time to recharge. Finding the time to establish a new routine in our lives may not be easy, but the results are always worth the time and effort.

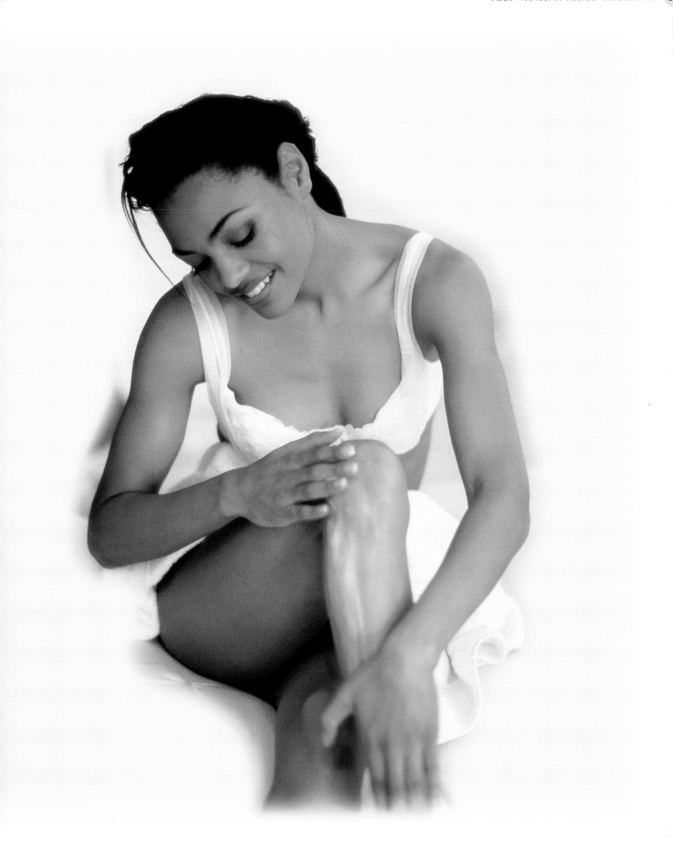

Breathing techniques

B*reathing is so natural, so fundamental to our existence, that most people take it for granted. However, if you suffer from asthma you'll know how precious air is and you may be more aware of your breathing than most people.*

It is estimated that one-quarter of people don't breathe as they should, a fact that can lead to all sorts of medical problems, not only asthma. In a relaxed state you should breathe roughly every six seconds, but if you have asthma you may be breathing much more often than that.

Hyperventilating, or breathing too much, can lead to chronic conditions such as headaches, tiredness, anxiety, irritable bowel syndrome, and even coronary heart disease.

How you breathe

Whether air enters the body through the nose or mouth, there are two basic ways of breathing: with the chest, or the top half of the lungs, and with the diaphragm, the umbrella-shaped muscle that separates the chest and abdomen.

In normal breathing, you draw air into the lungs, the diaphragm flattens, and the intercostal muscles between the ribs contract, so that the chest moves outward. As you breathe out, the diaphragm relaxes and resumes its dome shape, and the chest sinks. While your chest obviously moves in and out a little when you breathe, the main movement should be in the abdomen.

You tend to use the chest to breathe when you are excited, tense, or stressed. Instead of using the diaphragm, you use the muscles of the rib cage. But somehow, many people have gotten into the habit of using the chest too much, which means that they are living in a state of unnecessary heightened tension all the time.

Effective breathing

Relaxation is the key to good breathing and so is emotion—the more positive the emotion the better the breathing. Anxiety, fear, stress, and tension all quicken breathing and make it more shallow; pleasure, contentment, and emotional and physical well-being deepen and strengthen your breathing.

BREATHING OUT

Shallow breathing—when you inhale an inadequate amount of air, largely because you have not exhaled enough air—is common and can have harmful effects on the body. The key to avoiding shallow breathing is to concentrate on breathing out.
• *Breathe in through the nose and out through the mouth, sighing as you do so.*
• *Every time you sit down, breathe out long and slow. Aim for a count of five on every out breath.*
• *When you walk, count two on each in-breath and two on each out-breath. Gradually increase the count on each out breath to five.*

Both conventional and complementary medicine understand the importance of good breathing. But in some ancient systems it is the cornerstone of health. Indian holy men or yogis practice *pranayama*, or deep breathing, to calm the mind and spirit. In Traditional Chinese Medicine, harmony comes when your inner *qi* or life energy is at one with the *qi* in the air around you. ▶

Find out more	
Yoga	*90*
T'ai chi	*94*
Meditation	*100*

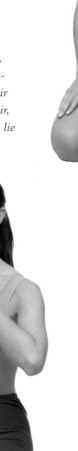

1 *Sit in a position that is comfortable. Some people are happy sitting cross-legged; others prefer sitting back on their heels. Alternatively, you can sit in a chair, preferably one with an upright back, or lie on a mat on the floor.*

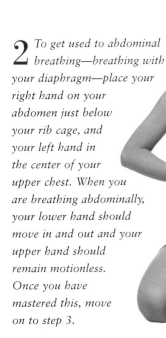

2 *To get used to abdominal breathing—breathing with your diaphragm—place your right hand on your abdomen just below your rib cage, and your left hand in the center of your upper chest. When you are breathing abdominally, your lower hand should move in and out and your upper hand should remain motionless. Once you have mastered this, move on to step 3.*

3 *Rest your hands in your lap one inside the other with thumbs lightly touching. Relax your shoulders—they should slope down and slightly backward when they are relaxed. Close your eyes or let them rest, unfocused. Breathe in deeply through your nose feeling your abdomen expand. Count to 10 as you breathe in, hold the breath for a few seconds, and slowly exhale letting out as much air as you can. As distractions slip into your mind, don't try to push them away or block them out. Let them float in and float out again, concentrating on your breathing. Repeat this 10 times.*

Breathing techniques

The key to the Buteyko method is measuring your control pause, the length of time you can manage without taking a breath.

THE BUTEYKO METHOD

Developed in the 1950s by a Russian scientist, Konstantin Buteyko, the Buteyko method is a series of exercises. The method is designed to retrain your breathing patterns. It is popular in Russia, Australia, New Zealand, and the UK, but almost unheard of elsewhere.

Buteyko theory

Practitioners believe that asthma is a breathing disorder, which develops because people with asthma hyperventilate, even during an attack. The normal intake of air is 7–10$\frac{1}{2}$ pints (4–6 liters) a minute. In a trial to test the technique in Brisbane, Australia, participants were breathing in 26$\frac{1}{2}$ pints (15 liters) a minute.

With each breath, you take in oxygen (O_2), which is absorbed into the blood. When you exhale you breathe out carbon dioxide (CO_2). The role of oxygen in breathing is clear, but CO_2 is often viewed simply as waste matter. However, you also need the right amount of CO_2 in the blood stream in order for oxygen to be transferred from the lungs to the blood and so to the vital organs. In this sense, CO_2 is vital for control of the major body systems such as the heart and circulatory, digestive, and immune systems. Carbon dioxide is stored in the alveoli in the lungs.

When you hyperventilate, you deplete your body of CO_2 by breathing out too much of it and diluting the amount retained in the alveoli. Because you do not have enough CO_2 in your blood, the red blood cells cannot release their oxygen. In simple terms, when you hyperventilate your body gets less oxygen, not more. Buteyko practitioners say this chronic hyperventilation causes conditions such as asthma and eczema.

Through the Buteyko method you can reprogram your breathing to prevent hyperventilation and so relieve your symptoms. If you know how to control your hyperventilation and normalize your breathing, you can overcome an attack and are well on the way to alleviating the symptoms of your asthma.

Practitioners of the Buteyko method maintain that after two or three days' treatment you will be able to cut your medication by 40 to 50 percent and after a few more days you should be able to reduce it by 80 to 100 percent.

The technique

The method—essentially a series of breathing exercises—looks too simple to be true. But many people who use it have dramatically reduced their medication and say that their symptoms have all but vanished.

Buteyko breathing exercises are actually complex and should be taught by a trained practitioner. You need to take between three and five classes lasting an hour and a half each, and these are expensive. If you don't see an improvement, however, Buteyko practitioners guarantee you your money back. Buteyko classes are held only in Russia, Australia, New Zealand, Israel, and the United Kingdom, but if you do not have access to them, the main elements of the method are described here.

The "control pause"

The course begins with what is called the control pause. This is the amount of time you can comfortably hold your breath and practitioners say that it will tell you whether you are overbreathing.

To measure your control pause sit comfortably in an upright chair, relax, and breathe out. Gently breathe in, then out again, holding your nose after you have breathed out. Hold your breath until you feel uncomfortable.

If you can hold your breath for a minute that is excellent, but a pause of 40–60 seconds shows that you are in good health. If you can hold your breath for 30 seconds you are mildly asthmatic and if it is around only 10 seconds you have severe asthma.

On the second day you continue with your control pause. Only those in the peak of health will be able to hold their breath for a minute, but if you fight the urge to breathe in you will find that each day your pause, whether it is 10 or 30 seconds, will get longer.

Adopt the routine of four long pauses and two medium ones, separated by three-minute intervals of shallow breathing, four times a day. Eventually your breathing will return to normal.
• Try to always breathe through your nose, not your mouth. This is fundamental to the Buteyko method. If your nose is blocked because of asthma, the breath-holding and shallow breathing exercises may be able to open it up.
• Don't lie down unless you are really sleepy, because lying down will increase your breathing. Sit upright in a chair to read, watch television, or meditate.
• Don't forget to take your asthma medication. Buteyko is not intended to exclude conventional medicine. Use your bronchodilator if, and only if, you feel tightness in your chest. If you want to adjust your steroid dose do so in consultation with your doctor.
• Focus on breathing less, not more. Stifle the desire to gulp at air.

Medical evidence

Despite the anecdotal success of the Buteyko method, many national asthma organizations remain skeptical, saying that they do not consider hyperventilation to be a factor in asthma.

However, clinical trials in Australia showed that people using the method cut their bronchodilator medication by 90 percent after six weeks and felt better. But there were no changes in the patients' peak flow rates, nor in routine tests to assess the severity of a patient's asthma.

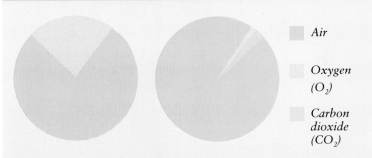

OXYGEN AND CARBON DIOXIDE

■ Air

■ Oxygen (O_2)

■ Carbon dioxide (CO_2)

Every lungful of air you take in consists of 20 percent oxygen and only 0.03 percent carbon dioxide (above left). But in order for there to be enough carbon dioxide to allow the transfer of oxygen from the lungs to the bloodstream—and so around the body—you need about 6 percent carbon dioxide and 2 percent oxygen in your lungs (above right). As a result, the body stores carbon dioxide in the alveoli, tiny air sacs in the lungs. Each lung contains more than 350 million alveoli, surrounded by blood capillaries.

Yoga

*A*n *ancient Hindu system of exercises or postures, called* asanas, *yoga unlocks tension and brings about physical, mental, and spiritual well-being. The word derives from the Sanskrit meaning "union."*

There are many different types of yoga, some of which have been practiced for more than 5,000 years. In the West, however, the most popular types are hatha yoga, which consists of a series of gentle exercises and postures, and iyengar yoga, which is more advanced and physically rigorous.

In addition to the postures, yoga incorporates meditation, breathing exercises (*pranayama*), relaxation, and diet. By practicing yoga regularly, not only do you tone your muscles, strengthen your spine, and become more supple, but you can also achieve a heightened awareness through control and discipline of your mind. Yoga was originally developed as a way of achieving heightened spirituality.

Yoga will help you to ease your asthma and allergies in all kinds of ways, by relieving stress and tension, and by regulating your breathing. It teaches you how to relax and not to panic and it will increase your strength and stamina.

Practitioners who teach yoga to people with asthma say that it can strengthen the respiratory muscles and tone the lung tissues. Learning breath control and relaxing the chest so that you breathe fully in and fully out will make your lungs less sensitive to allergens. If you practice yoga regularly you can see an improvement within weeks, not only for asthma but also for skin conditions such as eczema.

Yoga is not an exercise in the way that working out at the gym is (although your local fitness center may have yoga classes) nor is it something someone does to you, like acupuncture. It is a good idea to go to yoga classes to get used to the correct movements, but once you have grasped the postures yoga can be incorporated into your life and practiced quietly at home. The yoga asanas are designed to improve the flow of prana, or vital energy. The physical postures and, as important, the breathing exercises, calm the mind and improve the flow of "vital energy." Yoga is suitable for people of any age.

Yoga postures

There are around 80 postures, but most people practice only 20 or so. Wear loose clothing, with nothing on your feet. You cannot do yoga on a bed; you must work on a nonslip yoga mat or the floor.

Yoga should be practiced on an empty stomach, which is why many people do it when they wake up. Wait for three hours after a meal before you do your asanas and try to find a regular time, ideally before breakfast or your evening meal.

Classes usually start with stretching exercises and asanas are interspersed with deep relaxation and breathing exercises. They end with the corpse pose, a powerful yoga weapon against stress.

Never hurry or strain and if you can't do a full posture do as much as you can. Keep your movements slow and graceful and hold asanas for between 20 seconds and two minutes. In yoga it is important to do counter postures when you stretch:

bend backward after bending forward; stretch to the left after stretching to the right, and so on.

Work to your own limit, breathing slowly and holding for a few seconds. You may feel a bit of discomfort when you go into a stretch, but if you take it slowly, no harm should result.

Both postures and breathing exercises help respiratory disorders such as asthma, hay fever, bronchitis, sinusitis, colds, and coughs. People with asthma tend to have shallow breathing, and yoga deepens the breath and induces relaxation, dissipating any tension that might lead to an attack.

Start with a breathing exercise to calm and relax you. Yoga breathing exercises will help you develop good breathing habits and can alleviate your asthma or hay fever symptoms.

Alternate nostril breathing

Sit upright and place the thumb and index finger of your right hand on the bridge of your nose. Close your left nostril with the third finger. Breathe in through your open right nostril and breathe out vigorously and in spurts 10 times. Change hands and breathe through the other nostril.

Whispering breath

This exercise is recommended for anyone with a respiratory disorder, particularly asthma sufferers. Sit in front of a lighted candle with your hands, shoulders, and jaw relaxed. Breathe regularly. Inhale deeply and, through pouted lips, slowly blow at the candle. Do not blow it out, just make it flicker. When you have exhaled, close your mouth, breathe in through your nose, and repeat. ▶

Find out more	
Airways	289
Breathing techniques	86

Kapalabhati

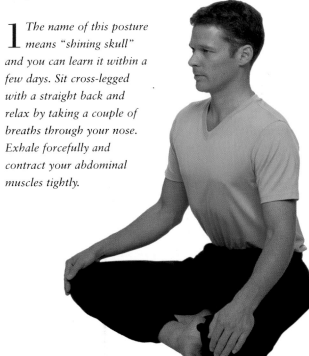

1 *The name of this posture means "shining skull" and you can learn it within a few days. Sit cross-legged with a straight back and relax by taking a couple of breaths through your nose. Exhale forcefully and contract your abdominal muscles tightly.*

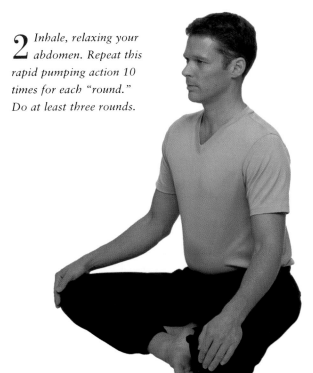

2 *Inhale, relaxing your abdomen. Repeat this rapid pumping action 10 times for each "round." Do at least three rounds.*

Yoga

The bow

1 *Lie on your stomach with your legs slightly apart and flat on the floor, and your arms by your sides, palms upward.*

2 *Breathing normally, bend your knees and bring them toward your buttocks. Slowly and carefully tilt your head backward and grasp your ankles with your hands.*

3 *Exhale and push your feet upward and away from you. Hold the posture for as long as you can, breathing regularly. Rest, then repeat.*

The triangle

1 *Stand up straight facing forward with your feet more than shoulder-width apart, with your right foot pointing to the right and your left turned in slightly. Extend your arms sideways at shoulder level, palms down.*

2 *Inhale, and as you exhale, bend to the right and slide your arm down your right leg, grasping as low down as you can. At the same time, move your left arm into the air.*

3 *Hold for several breaths, then repeat the exercise on the other side.*

The cobra

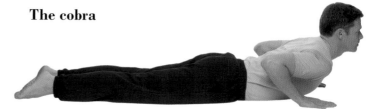

1 *Lie on your stomach with your forehead touching the floor, arms directly beneath your shoulders, and palms flat on the floor. Touch the floor with your chin, then your nose.*

2 *Inhale as you slowly arch backward. Keep your hips on the mat and don't strain.*

3 *Hold for as long as you can, breathing normally, then lower yourself to the start position. Rest, then repeat.*

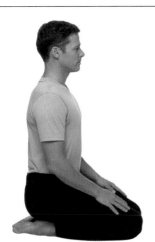

The camel

1 *Kneel, then sit on your heels with your toes outstretched. Rest your hands on your thighs.*

2 *Inhale and, without moving your feet or knees, lift your buttocks off your knees until you are kneeling upright.*

3 *Reach back and touch your left heel with your left hand. Allow your head to tilt backward.*

4 *Then reach back with your right hand to touch your right heel. Your arms, back, and legs should form as close to a rectangle as possible. Breathe normally, and hold for at least 10 seconds.*

Find out more

Managing your asthma	74
Choosing a therapy	82
Ayurvedic medicine	120

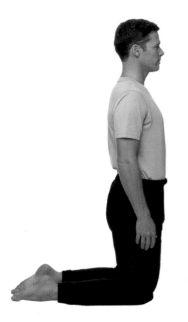

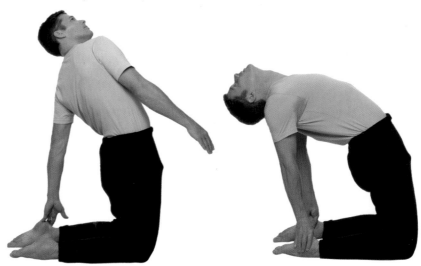

CASE HISTORY

Robert, now 50, brought his asthma under control through yoga. His asthma started when he was eight and he had it all through his childhood, teens, and twenties. He was allergic to pollen, molds, house dust mites, feathers, and certain foods. In his thirties he developed bronchitis from which he never fully recovered.

"Every year it seemed to get worse and worse. I was having regular asthma attacks and was taking more and more medication. Every night I would wake up in spasm and it was at that point that I met an Indian doctor who introduced me to yoga. I felt better almost immediately and over the course of about three

years, practicing yoga for about an hour and a half every day, I was completely cured. That was 20 years ago and I have had no medication since. I don't even get asthma in the pollen season.

I still practice yoga every day, though not as much as before. I don't like not to do any, but I can get by without it. Apart from curing my asthma, yoga has made me feel much more centered and able to cope with stress. Yoga doesn't cure everyone—I was lucky—but if you practice it regularly it will ease your symptoms. And you're empowering yourself—you are controlling your asthma, not the other way around."

T'ai chi

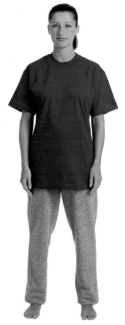

*W*hile most people rush to work, leaping out of bed and grabbing breakfast with only minutes to spare in their tight schedule, the Chinese start the day, often en masse, with beautiful dancelike movements called t'ai chi. At the crack of dawn, tens of millions of Chinese all over the world are practicing what was once described as "swimming on land."

T'ai chi, or t'ai chi chu'an (the three words mean "the supreme unity" and "fist"), looks like slow-motion walking. It is a series of gentle graceful movements flowing into one pattern, or form, designed to encourage the natural flow of energy, or *qi*, through the body's meridians, or energy channels. As long as qi is flowing freely, practitioners believe, you will be healthy.

T'ai chi—it is sometimes spelled taijiquan—is believed to have been developed around the 12th century by the Daoist mystic Chang San-Feng. He was forced by birth to join the army but was concerned about the hard and aggressive nature of the army's martial training, what we would today call kung fu.

He deserted the army and over the years developed the new dancelike movements to promote mental as well as physical development. Another legend has it that t'ai chi was developed as a martial art by monks, who were forbidden to carry any sort of weapon.

The exercises were inspired by the natural movements of nature—the wind, birds in flight, or the sea. It has been described as a nonviolent or "internal" martial art and this is an apt description.

While Westerners are competitive and taught to stretch themselves to the limit at work, at home, in exercise, and in their personal lives, t'ai chi emphasizes the power of flexibility, of yielding, and

"going with the flow."

Because t'ai chi is not competitive, it is usually practiced alone, though you can practice in pairs. There is one movement —"pushing hands"—which requires you to lead or push the hands of another person who has his or her eyes closed.

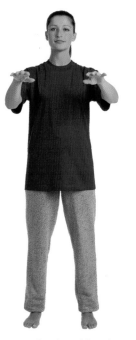

1 *Stand with your feet shoulder-width apart. Keep your knees unlocked.*

2 *With relaxed hands, breathe in and raise your arms to shoulder height.*

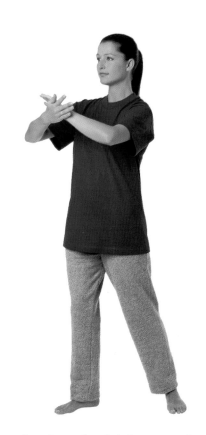

3 *Step forward and shift your weight onto your right foot. Cross your hands, the left hand in front with palm facing away from you and right palm facing you.*

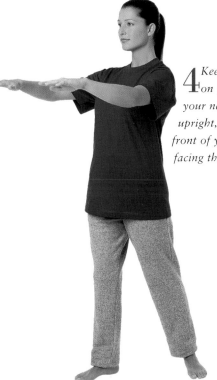

4 *Keeping your weight on your right foot and your neck and back upright, raise your arms in front of you with the palms facing the ground.*

5 *Shift your weight back onto the left foot. Bring your arms down toward you until the arms are at about waist height, with the palms facing downward.*

There are plenty of books and video courses to choose from, but t'ai chi is best learned through a class. Though the exercises are simple, the way they flow into one another is best demonstrated. The exercises illustrated here are intended to give you an idea of some of the basic movements. Wear loose clothing—a jogging suit is ideal—and flat shoes or leave your feet bare.

After warm-up exercises, your teacher will demonstrate the "short form," which consists of 37 movements that can be performed in about 10 minutes; the "long form" takes 20–40 minutes and has a total of 108 movements.

T'ai chi is difficult to learn at first because you have to remember the movements, but practice makes perfect and it gets easier with time. Like yoga, classes are quiet and unhurried and the teacher will explain the philosophy behind the movements. Each exercise begins and ends with standing still for a few seconds.

T'ai chi cannot be mastered in just a few weeks. It may take many months or even a year to gain a degree of proficiency. However, with a good teacher, you will start to experience subtle benefits after a few lessons.

T'ai chi, as part of Traditional Chinese Medicine (TCM), regards the mind, body, and spirit as one, all influencing one another. A positive change in one will influence the others. So the improved posture, relaxed muscles, and deep breathing needed to perform the movements will alleviate stress and stress-related ailments, such as tension headaches and anxiety. The concentration and discipline needed to remember the form strengthens the mind.

Always start your t'ai chi session with a series of warm-up exercises. Carrying out a few simple exercises ensures that your muscles and joints are loose before you start. It is best to perform t'ai chi in the open air, if possible.

6 *As you breathe out, push your arms forward, with the palms facing away from you, moving your weight back onto the right foot.*

CHAPTER FOUR

Qigong

Wu Chi

The Wu chi, or "emptiness," pose is the classic opening position for many qigong routines. Stand with knees slightly bent and feet shoulder-width apart and facing forward. Let your hands hang loosely at your sides and relax your shoulders. Stand for a few minutes feeling your abdomen expand and contract as you breathe in and out.

A n ancient Chinese system of movement, breathing, and meditation, qigong strengthens the qi. Qi means "vital essence" or "life-force" and gong means "work," so qigong is a discipline that allows you to gain control over your life-force.

Qigong (pronounced "chee gung") aims to maintain or restore balance and harmony of the mind and body. Through qigong, you can build up your *qi* and remove any blockages, which, according to Traditional Chinese Medicine (TCM), lead to disease.

The art of qigong is thousands of years old, but was suppressed during the Chinese Cultural Revolution (1965–76), possibly because of its close links with warfare. In China, warriors always built up their strength through practicing qigong. It made a comeback in the late 1970s and today more than 80 million Chinese practice qigong every day.

Practicing qigong lowers the heart rate and by doing so calms you and makes you breathe more efficiently. In qigong breathing, you breathe from the abdomen, not the chest. This diaphragmatic breathing not only tones

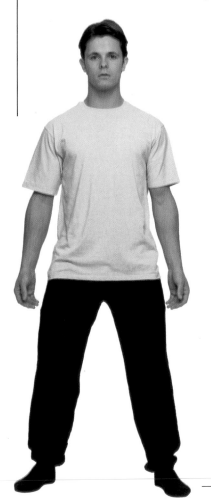

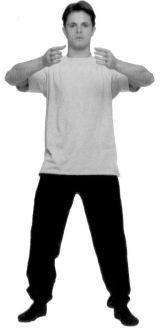

1 *Imagine you are holding a large ball in front of your chest. Raise your arms to slightly lower than shoulder height and bend your elbows to accommodate the ball. Hold this pose for a minute or two.*

2 *Raise your arms still further and turn your hands palm outward, with your fingers loose and slightly apart. Tilt your head back slightly so that you are looking through the space between your hands. Hold for a minute or two.*

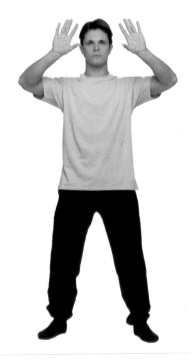

the abdominal muscles but also increases your lung capacity. Qigong is also believed to boost your immune system. A relaxation exercise known as Floating on the Ground is exactly the same as yoga's Corpse posture and is beneficial for anyone suffering from stress-related allergies.

Studies in China have shown that people who practice qigong regularly increase their forced vital capacity—the volume of air breathed out when exhaling forcefully—by over 16 percent. Practitioners also believe qigong increases the capacity to absorb oxygen.

It is best to be taught the exercises by a skilled practitioner, but once mastered, you can practice them yourself. Wear loose clothing, such as track pants and a T-shirt. Always be sure to exercise on an empty stomach.

Good posture, which enhances the flow of *qi*, is all-important in qigong. Knees are relaxed and slightly bent, the neck and shoulders relaxed and falling away—think of them lengthening and opening. The head should be light and free, balanced on the top of the spine, which should be straight but not stiff. You should be centered and stable, with your feet apart. Relax your abdomen, don't draw it in or stick your chest out. Your lips should be lightly touching, the mouth relaxed.

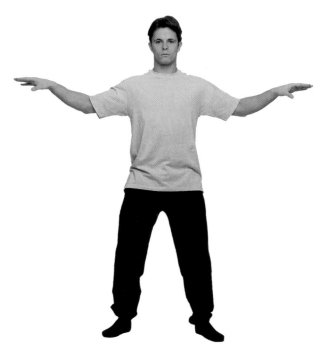

3 *Lower your arms, keeping your elbows bent, and extend them out to your sides, with your palms facing downward. Hold for a minute or two.*

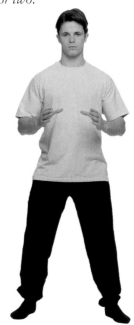

4 *Bring your hands to the front of your body, palms facing each other and fingers spread, as if you were holding a soccer ball in front of you. Hold for a minute or two.*

Autogenic training

Sometimes simply called autogenics or AT, autogenic training is a series of mental exercises that can bring about deep relaxation if practiced every day. This in turn promotes physical and mental well-being.

Autogenics works best if you are taught how to do it and then practice at home. In common with many complementary therapies, autogenics does not treat a specific ailment, but brings the body to a state in which its self-healing mechanisms are activated.

Derived from the Greek meaning "generated from within," autogenics was developed 75 years ago in Berlin by the German psychiatrist and neurologist Dr. Johannes Schultz. Using his knowledge of hypnosis, and influenced by the ideas and support of his colleague Sigmund Freud, he devised six silent verbal exercises. These were perfected by his followers, in particular by Dr. Wolfgang Luthe, who has popularized the training in the U.S. and Canada. AT is now practiced worldwide and there are two research centers—the Schultz Institute in Berlin and the Oskar Vogt Institute in Japan.

Autogenics is a mixture of self-hypnosis, positive affirmations, and deep relaxation. The principles consist of the repetition of the six standard exercises; a mental activity known as passive concentration in which you cultivate a relaxed attitude unconcerned with results; and the use of specific postures designed to avoid distractions.

If these are followed regularly and correctly, those who practice the training achieve an altered state of consciousness—the autogenic state—which is similar to the hypnotic state. Brain waves slow and there is an increase in alpha waves (characteristic of a brain at rest). Like all meditative techniques, autogenics allows you to turn your attention inward, switching off the "fight or flight" response and allowing your mind and body time to restore and repair themselves.

Visiting a practitioner

While you can practice autogenics by yourself, you need to be taught how to do it properly. Sessions may be one to one, or you may be part of a group of up to half a dozen people. You will be asked about your medical history and lifestyle, then asked to sit or lie down. Each exercise is aimed at relaxing a part of your body and achieving mental calm.

In the first exercise you concentrate on the heaviness of your limbs. You will be asked to lift your right arm and repeat silently, "My right arm is very heavy." You will repeat this with your other limbs. The second exercise focuses on the

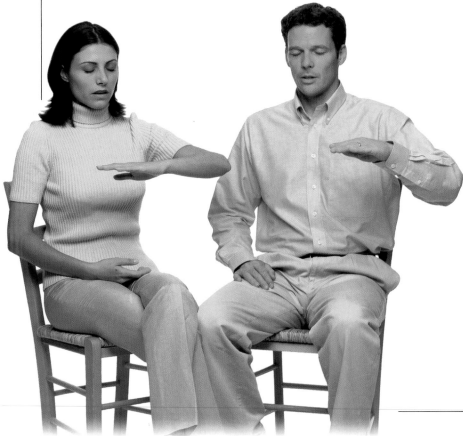

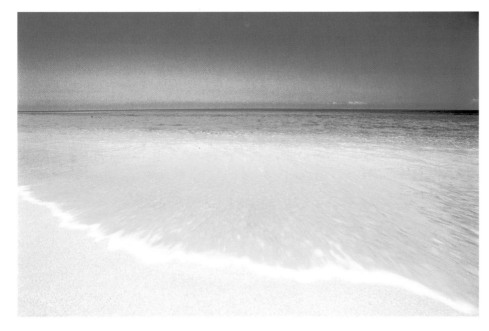

Find out more

Stress solutions	*58*
Self-hypnosis	*102*

To use visualization effectively, think of an image that suits your condition. An asthmatic, for example, may choose to be on a mountainside, breathing in clean air, while someone with itchy eczema may visualize bathing in a cool, crystal clear sea.

warmth in your limbs and you will say to yourself, "My arm is very warm." The third calms your heartbeat, the fourth relaxes the breath, the fifth warms the solar plexus, and the sixth cools the forehead. Through this repetition, you will reach the meditative state of passive concentration, in which your body's healing mechanisms are boosted.

Autogenic modification is a more advanced state of autogenic training and you may concentrate on particular parts of your body. Asthma sufferers, for example, might repeat, "My sinuses are cool and my chest is warm." The next stage is autogenic meditation in which you will be taught to use visualizations to accompany your inward repetitions.

Visualization

Harnessing the creative power of the imagination has been done for hundreds of years. St. Ignatius Loyola, in his book *Spiritual Exercises*, urged his followers to imagine events from the life of Christ in detail so as to become closer to God. The roots of visualization lie deep in magic, and ancient shamans or witch doctors were aware of the power of such techniques.

Visualization is similar to self-hypnosis and has links with autogenic training. The modern concept was developed in the 1970s as a branch of psychotherapy by the American cancer specialist Carl Simonton and his wife, Stephanie Matthews-Simonton, a psychologist. They used the discipline to help cancer patients who were asked to imagine their cancer being destroyed by their immune systems and treatments.

The Simontons maintained that their patients lived longer than patients who did not use visualization techniques and many cancer specialists have incorporated these techniques into cancer treatment. Visualization is now used for all sorts of reasons—to boost confidence, to prepare for a competitive activity such as athletics, to improve motivation, to release stress, and to fight illness.

Meditation

*P*ractised regularly, meditation aims to bring about total
relaxation and inner calm. Sitting quietly and breathing gently
sounds simple, but in fact meditation requires an inner discipline
you may initially find hard to achieve, but it is worth perservering.

The philosophy behind meditation is that, if you can sit still trying to exclude intrusive thoughts for about 20 minutes at a time, your mind is left free and automatically moves toward a greater feeling of happiness and fulfilment. When the mind is thus liberated it transcends the thinking process, leaving you in a state of complete inner quietness or bliss.

When you relax totally your blood pressure falls and your sense of health and well-being increases. Your breathing and pulse rates slow, your muscles relax, and levels of stress-linked chemicals and hormones fall. Even the electrical waves emitted by your brain change.

Many people with asthma and particular skin conditions, such as eczema, find it helps them. Scientific evidence from studies of transcendental meditation (TM), the best-studied form, backs this up. Research has shown that TM relaxes the muscles surrounding the airways. In one study in the early 1970s, 21 patients kept diaries of their meditation habits, asthma symptoms, medication, and general well-being over six months. At the end of the study, the patients had improved lung function and reported fewer symptoms. Most felt it had helped their asthma.

How to meditate

Ideally, you should meditate for 20 minutes twice a day, first thing in the morning and in the evening. You can teach yourself from books and videos, but it is easier to learn from a practitioner. You may find it difficult to bring the mind to stillness and the discipline of being in a group can be enormously beneficial. Many people find that it helps to focus on an object, such as a candle, or to repeat a mantra over and over again, as an aid to preventing their mind from wandering.

• Wear loose clothing and choose somewhere quiet to meditate. If you think you may be disturbed, unplug the telephone. Try to develop the habit of meditating at a particular time, so that it becomes part of your daily life, like brushing your teeth.

• The cross-legged lotus position is ideal, but you can also kneel with your feet tucked under your buttocks or sit astride

Wear comfortable clothing and meditate somewhere draft free that is neither too hot nor too cold. Closing your eyes will prevent stray thoughts from disturbing your sense of inner calm.

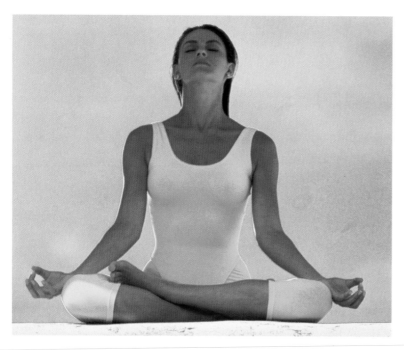

some cushions. If you feel uncomfortable on the floor, sit on an upright chair. Your shoulders should be relaxed, sloping slightly downward and backward. Your head should be drawn slightly back and your body weight should be directly over your hips. Your back should be straight, as if there is a string through your head, raising you up. Rest your hands lightly on your lap, with your thumbs touching, or on your thighs.

• Breathe deeply, remembering to breathe from your abdomen, filling your lungs and concentrating on the breath flowing in through your nose. Hold for a few seconds when your lungs are full, then slowly exhale. Repeat this 10 times.

• Continue breathing rhythmically, breathing through your nose. Focus on your mantra or object and if your mind wanders, don't get upset or annoyed. Just try to bring it back and refocus it on your mantra, image, or breathing.

• When you finish, don't jump up. Take your time and slowly become aware of your surroundings. Open your eyes, wait a minute, stretch, and return to normal consciousness.

Find out more

Yoga	90
Relaxation	102
Biofeedback	146

TYPES OF MEDITATION

BUDDHIST MEDITATION	Buddhist meditation has been practiced for thousands of years. You do not use a mantra; instead you concentrate on the "mindfulness of breathing" or "awareness of in-and-out breathing" (*anapani-sati*), and "development of loving kindness" (*metta-bhavana*) toward those around you.
TRANSCENDENTAL MEDITATION	Transcendental meditation, popularized in the 1960s by the Indian yogi Maharishi Mahesh, is increasingly practiced by professionals to alleviate stress and is gaining acceptance in medical circles. There are over four million people throughout the world who use TM. During a course you will be given a mantra, or meaningless word, the silent repetition of which induces deep relaxation.
MANTRA MEDITATION	This is a meditation on a simple word or phrase. You can choose your own or it can be given to you, as in TM. It can either mean something pleasurable to you, such as "love" or "peace" or it can be meaningless. The best-known mantra is "Om," which is the most sacred word for Hindus. You should repeat the mantra regularly and silently to yourself while you meditate.
CANDLE MEDITATION	You can meditate on a lighted candle, crystal, or icon. This is a yogic form of meditation known as *tratak*, in which you gaze at the object for about a minute, focusing on its texture, shape, and color, then close your eyes and visualize it. Ideally, it should be at eye level and about 3 ft (1 m) away. When the image fades, open your eyes and focus on the object again.
PRAYER	Repeating prayers with the help of a rosary is another form of meditation.

Relaxation and self-hypnosis

T*rue relaxation is difficult, but it is a skill well worth trying to learn. If your mind is not still, a lot of tension will remain in your body. It is important to learn to recognize when you are tense, as learning to relax may not only ease your asthma or allergy symptoms but also help you cope with an attack.*

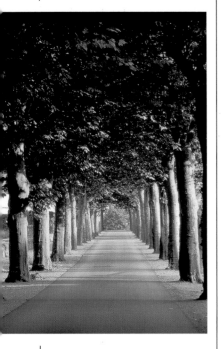

Many mental images can help you toward effective self-hypnosis, but those that work best usually involve a "counting" scene: a flight of stairs, a tree-lined avenue, or railroad tracks receding into the distance.

Relaxing is not about flopping down in front of the television or putting your feet up and enjoying a glass of wine, though both of those things can be pleasurable. Real relaxation is achieved by a profound letting go of your muscles, while your mind is alert but passive. Most people do not realize how tense they become sitting in front of a computer or even watching a favorite television program. But when you are under pressure your muscles tense, your shoulders ache and you may experience heart palpitations and shallow breathing.

There are plenty of simple things you can do to help you to relax: cutting down on stimulants such as tea, coffee, and tobacco, and switching to herbal teas, for example; scenting the air with calming essential oils, such as lavender; playing soothing relaxation tapes or music in the background. Your environment should induce feelings of contentment.

Devoting a short time each day to unwinding is not only relaxing but also wonderfully invigorating. You won't realize how tense you are until you feel your muscles slowly unwind. Wear loose clothing and relax on a mat on the floor, not the bed, where you might be tempted to fall asleep.

There is much similarity between deep relaxation and meditation. Several studies have shown that various kinds of meditation, yoga, and relaxation induced similar healthy benefits. Dr. Herbert Benson, founder of the Mind Body

Medical Institute at Harvard Medical School, has studied meditation and relaxation for 30 years and has identified a mental state, which he calls the relaxation response, that can reverse the damaging physical effects of stress.

This response may be brought about by meditation or Chinese postures, such as qigong and t'ai chi. But you do not have to learn ancient philosophies to relax. You can achieve relaxation by a simple exercise, a repetitive task, such as knitting or tapestry—or just sitting quietly and watching the sun go down. Whichever technique you use, it turns off what Dr. Benson calls "monkey mind"— the endless chatter that passes through your head like radio interference.

Your metabolism, heart rate, breathing, and brain waves slow down, your blood pressure falls, muscles relax, and your mind and body shift down a gear. When you relax and release tension your breathing automatically becomes more even and deeper.

Achieving the relaxation response

• Repeat a word or short phrase. It could be a secular word, such as ocean or love, or a religious word, such as Jesus or Allah, or a prayer.
• Sit quietly in a comfortable position and close your eyes.
• Breathe slowly and naturally, repeating your word or phrase.
• As everyday thoughts slip into your mind, brush them aside and return to

your repetition. Do not allow yourself to become anxious about how you are doing.

• Continue for 10 to 20 minutes and then slowly open your eyes. Wait for a few minutes before standing up.

• Practice this twice a day.

Self-hypnosis

This skill can be learned by anyone but it is best to be taught by a fully qualified hypnotherapist. You may decide that a course of hypnotherapy will help your allergies, and at the end of the treatment the hypnotherapist may teach you self-hypnosis to reinforce the suggestions he or she has made during the session.

These techniques are similar to those of autosuggestion and visualization, in which you imagine you are getting better and better every day. Some people are frightened they will lose control, become stuck in a hypnotic state, start exhibiting bizarre behavior, or be unable to respond to an emergency, such as a fire. But these concepts, however, are myths.

Throughout hypnosis, whether you are hypnotizing yourself, or whether you consult a hypnotherapist, you will remain in control and can come out of the hypnotic state at will. Far from being out of control, hypnotizing yourself is the highest form of self control, for you will be playing two roles—the hypnotist and the hypnotized.

• Lie down in a comfortable place—either on a sofa or the floor and breathe evenly, slowly becoming more relaxed.

• Imagine yourself walking down a long staircase or a tree-lined avenue, counting as you do so; with each step you take, you will go deeper and deeper into a trancelike state.

• Enjoy your deep relaxed state and repeat to yourself key statements, depending on your allergy. These autosuggestions can be accompanied by an image. If, for instance, your skin is hot and itchy, you could visualize yourself rolling in cool, wet grass.

• Intersperse these specific suggestions with positive thoughts, such as "I feel full of health" or "Every day, my symptoms are getting better and better."

• When you feel ready to come out of your hypnotic state, reverse the image that you used to take you there. So walk back down the tree-lined avenue to the gate, open it, and release yourself, counting down from 10 to zero.

Find out more

Stress solutions	*58*
Meditation	*100*

Relaxation involves learning to ban thoughts that aggravate stress levels. Lying comfortably listening to music can help you to tune out troubling thoughts, bringing benefits to both mind and body.

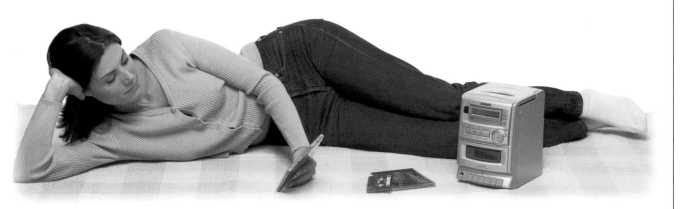

Aromatherapy

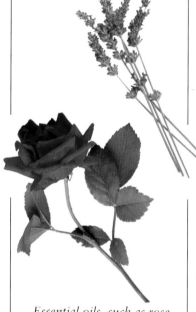

Gloriously relaxing, aromatherapy is good for stress-related conditions, such as migraine, anxiety, and insomnia. Digestive problems also respond well, as do muscular aches and pains, premenstrual syndrome, painful periods, and menopausal problems. Aromatherapists say it is good for the skin as well.

The power of perfumed oils to soothe and heal has been known for thousands of years across many cultures. A French chemist, René-Maurice Gattefossé, who studied the healing properties of plant oils, first used the word "aromatherapy" in the 1920s.

There are around 400 plant essences and each is believed to have a particular healing property. Essential oils are extracted from the flowers, leaves, seeds, roots, and stalks of aromatic plants and trees by steam distillation. The oils are highly concentrated and it may take hundreds of pounds of a plant to make just one gallon of essential oil, which means the oils are expensive and sold in tiny amounts, usually in small glass bottles.

Essential oils are massaged into the skin or inhaled in an infusion or sprinkled in a bath. The oils enter the bloodstream either through the skin or the nose, and work with nature to bring about healing.

How oils work

Essential oils work in two ways. When they are massaged into the skin, they reach the blood stream rapidly, and studies show they begin to have a healing effect in about 20 minutes. A full body massage will get the oil into the system faster than inhaling does.

In addition, their heady perfume stimulates the sense of smell, which in turn affects part of the brain called the limbic system, home of moods and emotions. Smell is the most primitive sense and most people know that long-since-forgotten smells, if reencountered, can bring back a flood of memories.

Visiting an aromatherapist

Aromatherapy can be practiced at home, but it may be advisable to consult a professional. On the first visit you will be asked about your medical history and lifestyle. Pure essential oils should never be applied directly to the skin. Because they are pure, they are potent, so the therapist will mix a few drops with a teaspoon of carrier oil, such as grapeseed or almond. The therapist will either select oils that are right for you or ask you to make your own choice.

The massage is based on Swedish techniques and will stimulate the circulatory and lymphatic systems and loosen tense muscles. Afterward, you should feel totally relaxed. You will not reek of perfume because all of it will have been absorbed, nor will you be greasy, for all the oil will have been massaged in.

Using oils

Apart from being used for massages, oils can be added to bath water—5 drops in warm water should be enough. You can also make a soothing inhalation by putting 3–4 drops in a bowl of hot water. Cover your head with a towel and breathe in the vapor for about 5 minutes.

Essential oils, such as rose and lavender, are distilled from many parts of the plant, including the leaves and flowers.

A vaporizer gently warms an essential oil to release its aroma into the air.

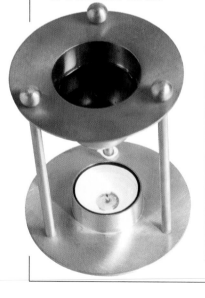

USEFUL ESSENTIAL OILS

ESSENTIAL OIL	USES
CAJUPUT	Respiratory infections, including colds, coughs, sinus infections, and sore throats
CHAMOMILE	Allergies, stomach and menstrual cramps, skin irritation or inflammation
CINNAMON	Tones the circulatory, respiratory, and digestive systems
CITRONELLA	An effective insect repellent
GERANIUM	Soothes the skin and is suitable for dry, oily, or problem skin
GINGER	Strengthens the immune system, also good for indigestion, nausea
LAVENDER	Bites and stings, burns, eczema, dermatitis, asthma, immune deficiency, insomnia
MELISSA	Stress, migraines, and nervous asthma
MYRRH	Chronic respiratory conditions, mouth and throat infections
PEPPERMINT	Nausea, indigestion, diarrhea, gas, bloating, headache, sinus congestion
ROSE	Anxiety and depression, stress, menstrual disorders, skin care, particularly more mature skin
SANDALWOOD	Urinary and throat infections, stress, immune deficiency, dry skin
TEA TREE	Respiratory and skin infections, insect bites and stings, coughs, colds, phlegm, gynecological problems

Warning

• Never swallow essential oils—they can be lethal. Keep them out of reach of children.

• Never use pure essential oils near your eyes.

• Some citrus oils, in combination with sunlight, are phototoxic, that is they sensitize the skin to light. You should not apply the following oils to your skin if you are about to sun bathe or use a sunbed: verbena, bergamot, orange, lemon, or any other citrus oil. If you do, you may burn in patches, and these patches may never go away.

• If you are pregnant, consult a qualified aromatherapist—some oils are not suitable.

• If you have severe asthma, do not have an aromatherapy massage without consulting your doctor.

• If you have high blood pressure, diabetes, epilepsy, or a skin irritation, such as contact dermatitis, consult an aromatherapist before using any essential oil.

Practitioner-administered therapies

If you are suffering from a long-standing and possibly severe condition, such as asthma, eczema, or celiac disease, it's wise to visit a practitioner so he or she can not only see your symptoms but also make an accurate diagnosis of what is wrong.

Conventional doctors tend to focus on your illness, but complementary medicine is holistic, and a complementary practitioner will pay just as much attention to your mental, emotional, and spiritual state as to your symptoms. Complementary practitioners want to find the reason why you became ill in the first place. A practitioner will, therefore, ask you all kinds of questions about your emotional life, work, diet, and sleeping habits—subjects that few doctors touch on. This is because all complementary therapies, but particularly those administered by practitioners, are founded on two theories. The first is that given the right set of circumstances, such as a good diet, a clean environment, fresh air, and exercise, the body has a tendency toward "homeostatis" or good health. The second concept is one of energy, which lies at the heart of most complementary therapies. In Traditional Chinese Medicine it is called *qi*, in Japanese medicine it is *ki*, and in Hindu philosophy it is *prana*. Homeopaths talk of a "vital force" as do naturopaths. A complementary practitioner will assess the state of your energy and if it is "stagnant" or "blocked" restore it to healthy levels by manipulation, a massage, or by using needles.

Western medicine only recognizes this energy on a physical level, but scientists have discovered that it can be manipulated and passed from one person to another. This may be the explanation behind therapies that defy logical explanation, such as healing.

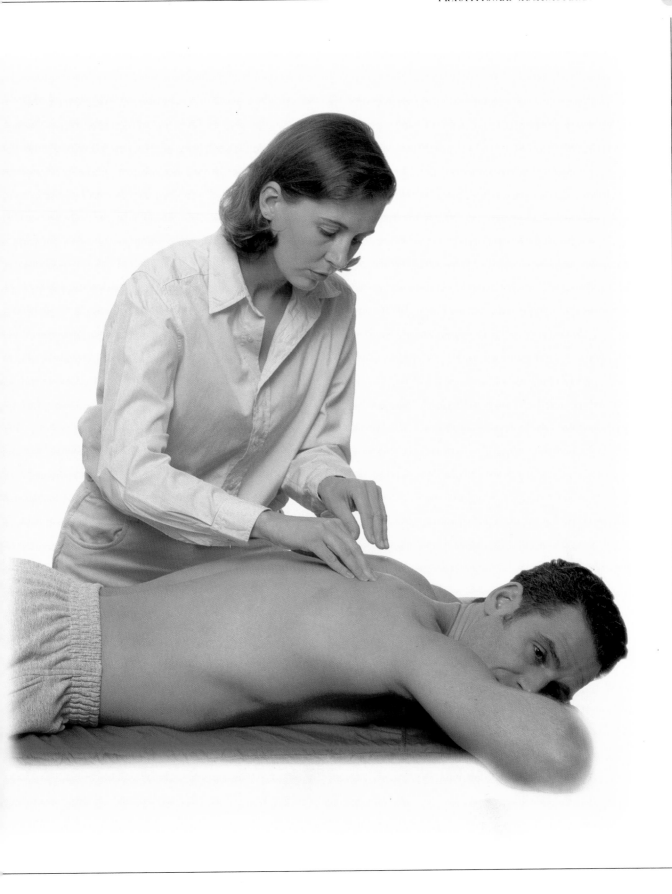

CHAPTER FOUR

Acupuncture and acupressure

O*ne of a number of treatments used in Traditional Chinese Medicine (TCM), acupressure involves applying pressure to precise points on the body to improve the flow of* qi, *or vital energy. Acupuncture applies needles to the same points.*

The first medical textbook written on acupuncture was *The Yellow Emperor's Classic of Internal Medicine (Nei Jing)* published between 300 and 100 BC, but there is archaeological evidence that acupuncture has been practiced in China for at least 3,500 years. It is still practiced there alongside conventional medicine and is increasingly popular in the West.

The philosophy behind TCM

An orthodox doctor may concentrate on the diseased or ailing part of the body, but a practitioner of TCM views a patient holistically, taking into account his or her physical, emotional, and mental states, as well as specific aches and pains.

In Chinese medicine, the body is believed to possess a network of invisible pathways called meridians, along which courses *qi*, a form of energy, vital force, or subtle breath. The concept of a vital energy pervading all things is fundamental to many Oriental systems of medicine, which maintain that as long as this energy flows freely, you remain healthy. When the energy becomes sluggish or stagnant, blocking the meridians, you fall ill. For perfect health you should be mentally and physically in harmony. Emotional as well as physical disturbances create disharmonies in the body.

Equally important is the belief that the *qi* should not only be balanced in your body but it should also be in harmony with the energies in the universe. This means that you are in harmony with nature and in tune with the seasons.

In common with other Oriental therapies, acupuncture aims to stimulate the release of energy and restore balance to the system by unblocking the meridians. In acupuncture this is done through placing needles in specific points along the meridians; in other therapies it is achieved through finger pressure or body massage. There are 365 acupoints on the body.

Qi itself is only strong—signifying a healthy individual—if yin and yang, two opposing forces, are balanced in the body. Yin represents the shady side of the mountain and symbolizes darkness, passivity, coldness, dampness, inferiority, and negativity; yang is the sunny side of the mountain and signifies heat, light, activity, the positive, and expressiveness.

By inserting fine needles at specific points, an acupuncturist aims to restore the body's flow of energy to its natural, healthy state.

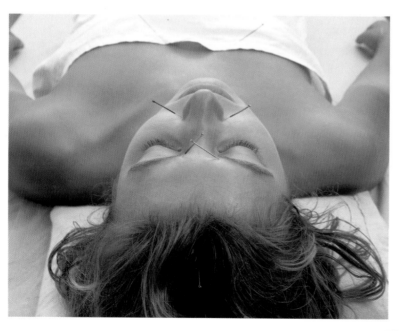

MOXIBUSTION

Moxibustion is used to warm your qi and may be chosen if you are deficient in yang. The technique involves placing a small cone, or moxa, of mugwort—sometimes also with a slice of ginger—over the acupuncture point. The cone is lit and allowed to smoulder until the skin is warm. This is repeated several times on the same point. Alternatively, the tip of a moxa stick may be lit and held above the skin over the acupuncture point.

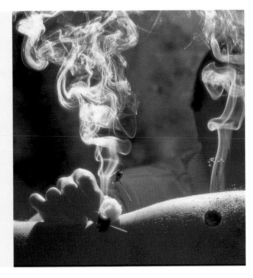

One of the main tasks of a practitioner of TCM is to observe the relationship between yin and yang and make adjustments to bring about harmony.

Visiting an acupuncturist

Your first session will take about an hour and the practitioner will take notes of your symptoms, medical history, lifestyle, and diet. Don't exercise, eat a large meal, drink alcohol, or have a shower or bath immediately before or after an acupuncture session.

To diagnose your illness, acupuncturists use the four classic Chinese examinations—touching, looking, smelling, and asking. The sheen of your hair, the brightness of your eyes, and the pallor of your skin are as important as your medical history. Your tongue will be examined: if you are healthy it should be pink and moist with little or no coating.

The acupuncturist will also take your pulse at both wrists. There are six pulses in each wrist (corresponding to the meridians) and they can have up to 28 qualities. The acupuncturist will then ask you to lie comfortably on a couch and he or she will place the needles in certain points along the chosen meridians. The acupuncturist will manipulate the needles and they may be removed immediately or left in for some minutes. There have been reports of skin irritation caused by needles and of bleeding when the needles are withdrawn.

There is good evidence that acupuncture can relieve asthma symptoms and build up defense against allergies. Many practitioners say that they have an 80 percent success rate in clearing up skin conditions such as eczema. ▶

ACUPUNCTURE NEEDLES

Acupuncture needles are stainless steel, usually disposable, and tipped with steel or copper. They vary in length and are so fine that you shouldn't feel discomfort when they are inserted. Needles can be inserted up to 4 inches (12 cm) deep if necessary. Because acupuncture points are usually close to the bone, the deeper the bone, the further the needle has to go. The acupuncturist may remove the needle instantly or leave it for up to 20 minutes, sometimes flicking or twirling it. If the needles are inserted correctly, it shouldn't be painful, but you may find it uncomfortable.

Acupuncture and acupressure

Acupressure

Acupuncture without the needles, acupressure involves a practitioner using his or her fingers, thumbs, hands, feet, and elbows to stimulate the acupoints and bring about health and well-being.

Acupressure is common in Asia and is gaining in popularity in the West. The techniques vary from country to country so there are several versions being practiced. A full Chinese acupressure massage, for example, is called tuina; a similar Japanese massage is called shiatsu. The oldest system is shen tao, in which the practitioner applies light pressure with the fingertips. All acupressure massages, however, are concerned with stimulating the energy in the body by pressing the acupoints, which act as valves for *qi*.

Musculoskeletal disorders, stress, digestive disorders, depression, anxiety, migraine, and irritable bowel syndrome, as well as allergies and emotional problems, can all benefit from acupressure. Pressure on the acupoints stimulates the immune system and promotes the release of endorphins, the body's natural painkillers.

You will usually be asked to lie down for a shiatsu massage for asthma. The treatment may begin with the practitioner placing one hand on your breast bone, between the nipples, and the other just below your navel.

Self-treatment with acupressure

• To stop nausea press a point 2 inches (5 cm) below the wrist crease, between the two tendons. This stops postoperative vomiting and nausea after chemotherapy.
• To lessen an allergic reaction, stretch out your arm and press the crease on the inside of your elbow. Or bend your arm and place your thumb at the end of the elbow crease on the inside. Once you have located this spot, stretch your arm out and stimulate the point.

Shiatsu

From the Japanese word meaning "finger massage," shiatsu works by stimulating the body's vital force, *qi* (or *ki*), which flows through the body's meridians.

Although it has developed in Japan in the 20th century, shiatsu has its roots in an ancient Japanese form of massage called *anma*, which consisted of pressing and rubbing the feet and hands with the fingers and palms of the hand. It was originally used to treat specific conditions, but it gradually developed into a form of pleasurable relaxation. Shiatsu is now used alongside Western medicine in Japan.

A shiatsu practitioner applies pressure to the acupoints—*tsubos* in Japanese—to rebalance the *ki* to promote health and treat specific conditions. The *ki* can be overactive, or blocked (*jitsu*), or depleted (*kyo*), all of which can result in lack of energy and ill-health. The practitioner aims to balance the body's *jitsu* and *kyo*.

Shiatsu is good for musculoskeletal problems, particularly in the lower back and neck, because it eases muscular tension and stiffness. It helps stimulate the circulation. It is reputed to be particularly good for asthma, as well as anxiety, rheumatism, insomnia, painful menstruation, depression, and fatigue.

Visiting a practitioner

On the day of your session, avoid alcohol, eat lightly, and don't take a shower or long, hot bath. You will remain clothed so wear loose garments, preferably cotton. Shiatsu practitioners work on the floor, usually on a mat or futon.

The practitioner will use the Oriental "four methods" of diagnosis—listening, observing, touching, and smelling—and ask about your work, home life, diet, and illnesses, past or present, and may take your pulse in the traditional Chinese way. By gently pressing the *hara* in the lower abdomen, he or she will assess the flow of *ki* in the meridians and internal organs.

Treatment is given in four ways: stretching and squeezing to break up the energy blockages; pressing the body at right angles, sometimes with the knee or elbow, to increase the blood flow; rocking to counteract agitations in the energy flow; and gently holding along the meridians or on specific points to enhance the flow of energy.

The practitioner may use thumbs, fingers, palms, elbows, knees, and feet to apply pressure and sometimes gentle stretches are incorporated. Shiatsu is not painful, but some of the acupoints where the energy is blocked may feel tender.

At the end of the session, you should feel invigorated yet relaxed. There may also be "healing" reactions for a day, as toxins and emotions are released.

Pressure on the point Lu 1—between the chest and shoulder—is of great benefit for the lungs (below left). A practitioner may also stretch your body to open the lung meridian, and apply pressure along the inner arm (below).

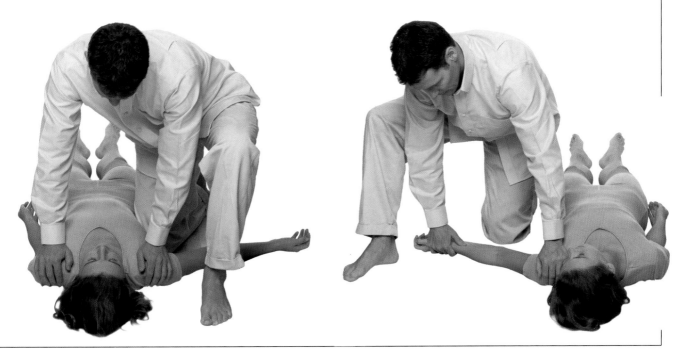

Chinese herbal medicine

Conventional medicine can sometimes cure some serious diseases, such as cancer, but against a chronic condition like eczema it is less effective. It can keep the symptoms at bay, but often at a cost in terms of side effects. If you have eczema on your face, where the use of topical steroids is not recommended, conventional medicine offers little.

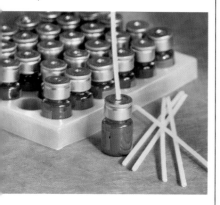

Chinese herbal remedies come in a variety of forms, including tinctures, pills, powders, and herbs.

Every culture and race has had its own form of herbal medicine. Physical evidence of humans using herbs goes back 60,000 years to a Neanderthal burial site uncovered in 1960.

Chinese herbal medicine is part of Traditional Chinese Medicine (TCM) and has been practiced for over 5,000 years. Just as an acupuncturist will try to stimulate the *qi* with needles, the medical herbalist will do the same with herbs, and each herb is said to go to a certain meridian, part of the invisible network along which the *qi* moves. Some herbs will tone and strengthen the *qi*; others will help it to move better.

The *Nei Jing* (*The Yellow Emperor's Classic of Internal Medicine*), written almost 2,500 years ago, is the earliest and most important document outlining the principles of TCM. It takes the form of a conversation between the Yellow Emperor and his minister Qi Bo on the subject of medicine and outlines the theories of yin and yang, meridians and the five elements. Even now in China it is seen as fundamental to the study of medicine.

Some of the earliest descriptions of herbal remedies in China date from the third century and are found in *Shen Nong Bencaojing* (*Classic of Roots and Herbs of Shen Nong*). It records the story of the Emperor Yen (Shen Nong), who tasted various herbs—even the poisonous ones— and passed his findings down verbally from generation to generation.

In modern China, TCM and Western medicine coexist, and TCM hospitals have departments specializing in Western medicine and vice versa. Some doctors are qualified in both and practice both.

Extensive research has been carried out on Chinese herbal medicine in China and its practitioners claim that it is

TREATING CHILDREN

Children and babies can be given Chinese herbal medicine. Because babies are very sensitive to medicine, their condition may improve dramatically with small doses of herbs. Practitioners should therefore see them frequently to monitor their progress. Children over the age of one year may be given herbal mixtures sweetened with honey.

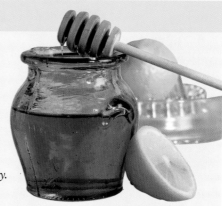

excellent for digestive complaints such as irritable bowel syndrome; respiratory diseases, such as chronic bronchitis, allergic rhinitis and asthma; and conditions such as chronic fatigue syndrome. There are herbs that eliminate toxins, as well as many tonics that are missing from modern medicines.

Chinese herbal medicine has proved to be very effective for beating eczema, with the added benefit of few or no side effects. Following reports about the success in tackling skin conditions of a Chinese doctor in London's Chinatown, the head of dermatology at London's Royal Free Hospital undertook a study of 37 children with severe and disabling atopic eczema. Each was given a mixture of 10 Chinese herbs whose formula had been devised by the Chinese practitioner, Dr. Ding-Hui Lou.

Of these children, 60 percent showed significant improvement and there were no adverse side effects. The same mixture was also used on adults with dermatitis, some of whom had suffered for years, and they too showed an improvement. Small wonder that Chinese herbal medicine is growing in popularity in the West, and many people afflicted with chronic ailments are actively searching out practitioners.

Visiting a practitioner

Your first session will take about an hour and you will be diagnosed in the traditional four ways—observing, listening, smelling, and touching.

The practitioner will ask you about your symptoms, medical history, lifestyle, and diet, and will want to know details such as whether you are anxious, tense, or stressed. He will look at the color of your complexion, your posture, check

your tongue, listen to your voice, and ask questions about whether you feel chilly, sweat a lot, or have headaches or aches and pains. As always in a TCM diagnosis, the practitioner will take your pulse at both wrists.

Once the practitioner has diagnosed your condition, he or she will make up a mixture of herbs for you. There are 3,500 Chinese herbal products, all of which are imported either from China or Hong Kong. Most practitioners use around 300 herbs. These aren't the sort of dried herbs that you keep on a kitchen shelf. You may get a large bag containing 10 to 15 herbs, seeds, bark, flowers, fruit, roots, and minerals mixed together.

From this you will prepare a *tang*, a tea made from boiling and reboiling the herbs. You will drink the resulting liquid a couple of times a day, usually before a meal, for the next few days. It has its own distinctive flavor, which some people find quite pleasant and others deem to be unpalatable.

Each herb has a particular function and the herbs act in concert to restore you to health and well-being. Finding the exact combination is an art that is difficult to achieve, and in China they say it takes 50 years to become a master herbalist. The practitioner may also prescribe remedies as pills, tonics, pastes, ointments, creams, and lotions.

The aim of the herbalist is to strengthen your *qi*, and use that internal strength to make the body better able to withstand external factors, such as viruses and bacteria. In the Western medical system this would be called strengthening the immune system. ▶

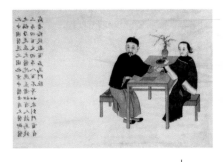

Pulse-taking in TCM is a subtle and sophisticated diagnostic skill. It is far more complex than in Western medicine.

Most Chinese remedies, such as ginseng, are derived from plants, but others are of mineral or animal origin.

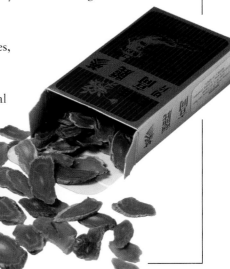

CHAPTER FOUR

Chinese herbal medicine

Chinese herbal remedies are made into formulas prescribed by practitioners to suit the individual needs of each patient.

Asthma

In Chinese medicine, asthma is seen as a disruption of *qi* caused by too much "phlegm" production, which can be brought about by a variety of factors, but is often due to a weakness of the kidneys, lungs, and spleen. ("Phlegm" in TCM refers to a disharmony in the body fluids that can block both physical and

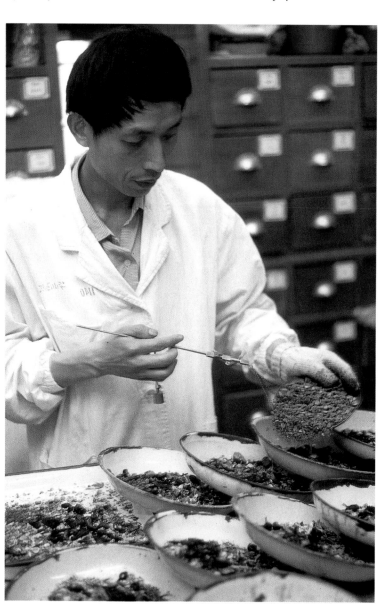

emotional functions. It is not the same as phlegm in the Western sense.) The practitioner may prescribe a kidney, lung, or spleen tonic. Ephedra and bitter almond seed help stop wheezing. (Ephedra, however, can be dangerous and should be taken only under supervision from a doctor or qualified herbalist.)

Too much "phlegm" can also be caused by a poor diet with too many "sticky" foods, such as chocolate, cheese, milk, and other dairy products. Eating irregularly also increases "phlegm" production.

Eczema

This condition is associated with the lungs, stomach, heart, and blood. According to TCM practitioners there are various types of eczema. One is where the skin is itchy, hot, and weeping; another is caused by heat in the blood, and your skin is dry, red, and itchy. A third kind is caused by "wind," and the skin erupts into blisters. The treatment is tailored according to which kind of eczema you have. Oriental wormwood or Chinese gentian, peony root and *Rumania* are used for the type caused by "wind."

Anxiety

In TCM, anxiety is often seen as an imbalance of the spleen and liver. Chinese angelica and ginseng may be used to strengthen the spleen and move energy through the liver.

CHINESE TONIC HERBS

Ginseng

This "king" of tonic herbs comes in two types—red, or Korean, ginseng and white ginseng. The latter is used as a general tonic for fatigue and weakness and can help insomnia. Red ginseng is a powerful

PRECAUTIONS WITH CHINESE HERBS

It is important to visit a reputable practitioner, who is fully qualified to prescribe and supply herbs. It is also advisable to make sure that the practitioner you visit belongs to a bona fide organization. Never buy herbal remedies by mail order and only buy an herbal remedy if the package clearly states what it contains. This will ensure that:

• The herbal products that are used are authentic and uncontaminated. Chinese herbs have been known to contain poisonous metals, such as lead, and/or conventional drugs, such as paracetamol.

• The herbs are not adulterated with animal products from endangered species, such as rhino horn, tiger bone, and bile from bears. This practice is now illegal and reputable practitioners do not stock the products of endangered species.

Note Seek medical advice before taking Chinese herbs if you are pregnant or have had liver disease in the past. If you feel unwell, stop taking the herbs or tablets immediately, tell the practitioner who dispensed the herbs, and tell your doctor.

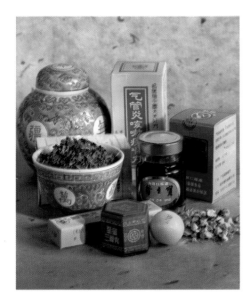

Different herbs are classified as cold, cool, warm, hot, or neutral depending on the way in which they alter the balance of qi within the body. The taste and smell of an herb is also important.

tonic. It is good for colds, poor circulation, and breathlessness. It can also be used in emergencies to treat shock.

Scientific studies suggest that ginseng stimulates the natural killer cells in the immune system and may also boost brain function. Although ginseng is widely available, you are recommended to consult a qualified practitioner. You should not take ginseng if you suffer from palpitations, high blood pressure, or frequent headaches.

Ginger

This root affects the stomach, spleen, and lung meridians and is used to treat nausea and vomiting and the common cold, and to detoxify the body. It may also be used as a medium in moxibustion, when moxa is placed on a slice of ginger laid on the skin, and burned down to the ginger slice.

Ginger is used for its warming properties. In addition to its use as a food, it can be made into a hot poultice and applied directly to expel cold from the internal organs.

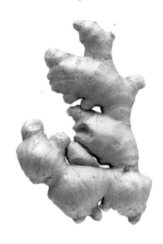

Western herbal medicine

*T*he use of herbs, flowers, and plants to cure and heal is the most ancient form of medicine. It is found in all parts of the world and is often handed down from generation to generation. As early as 450 BC, Hippocrates, the "father of modern medicine," was recommending senna as a laxative and it is still being prescribed today.

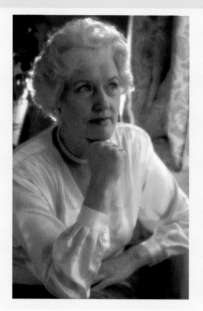

The flower, leaf, stem, root, or seeds of a plant may have medicinal properties.

In medieval times herbalism was surrounded by superstitious practices and linked to witchcraft, so it was criticized by the church. But it flourished in China, India, and South America, and when European immigrants landed in America, they added Native North American remedies to their own pool of herbal knowledge and herbal schools were established. In 1653 Nicholas Culpeper published his *English Physician and Complete Herbal*, the first book on herbalism in the English language.

Until a century ago, all medicines were derived from plants. But as modern medicine and the manufacture of synthetic drugs grew, herbalism fell out of favor and was dismissed as "folk" medicine. Yet many modern drugs are based on plant remedies. The best known example is aspirin, a synthetic drug based on the components of willow tree bark.

There are thousands of plants and herbs a practitioner can choose from, but most use about 200. These are described according to their effect or action on the body—in other words, what they make the body do. Some, like witch hazel, have astringent properties, others, like valerian, have sedative qualities, while others, such

CASE HISTORY

Mary, 60, has had asthma since she was 20, but found that reliever medication made her cough badly, though she still felt she had to take it. She kept her symptoms in check with steroids, but she found that she was having to take more and more of the drug to manage her asthma. She knew she was at an age when her asthma would only get worse.

"I was having a very bad time when I just couldn't control it. My daughter-in-law, a nurse, suggested I visit an herbalist, so I thought I would give it a try. The herbalist is always very thorough. She checks my blood pressure, listens to my chest, and talks to me before making up a batch of medicine for me. She varies the mixture depending on my health. I take a teaspoon of the mixture in warm water three times a day.

I'm sure it has had some effect. I feel much stronger and don't get out of breath as easily. I haven't cut down on my steroid medication, but I don't take any reliever now. I used to have to use it, even though it made me cough. Herbal medicine complements my drugs regime—I'm too severe an asthmatic for it to take the place of medication."

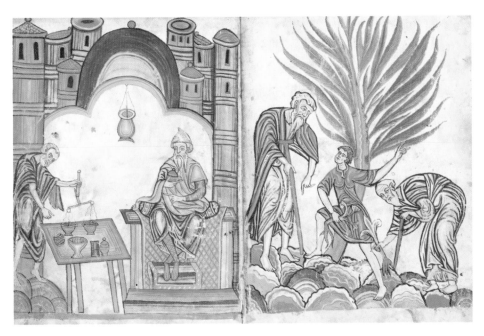

Before the development of modern laboratory-manufactured drugs, almost all medicines were derived from natural herbal sources.

as gentian, stimulate the digestion.

Your remedy may contain a dozen herbs and may work within a few days, although chronic conditions take longer to treat. You should see some improvement in your symptoms after a few weeks. It is likely that the herbalist will advise you on your diet, and will recommend you include fresh fruit, vegetables, and wholefoods in your diet.

Herbal medicine may be used to treat any condition but is particularly good for skin complaints such as chronic eczema and psoriasis, stress-related conditions such as migraines, digestive disorders such as irritable bowel syndrome, and respiratory infections, sore throats, and colds. Many herbal remedies are prescribed in order to clean out or detoxify the body.

While a manufactured drug may contain the same main constituent as a plant, for instance, some heart medications are made from digitalis,

which comes from the foxglove, it will have side effects. Herbalists claim that remedies that use the whole plant will not produce side effects because the other parts of the plant contain substances that will balance the more potent constituents. Modern pharmaceutical drugs contain only one component.

Visiting a practitioner

Your first session will be the longest—around an hour—and the herbalist will ask you details about your medical history, diet, work, emotional and mental state, and lifestyle. He or she may focus on whether you have any stress in your life.

Herbalists are trained in Western medical diagnosis, so your practitioner will take your pulse and blood pressure, check the glands in your neck, and sound your chest with a stethoscope, just like a conventional doctor. ▶

Plant remedies may be prepared as creams and ointments, which you apply externally. They are absorbed through the skin and enter the bloodstream.

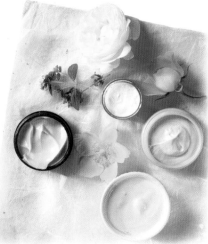

CHAPTER FOUR

Western herbal medicine

Types of herbal remedy

Herbs can be prescribed in several ways:
- Pills, capsules, and powders
- Teas and tisanes
- Tinctures—concentrated extracts of herbs in a water and alcohol solvent
- Syrups—the herb is boiled in water, and sugar is added as a preservative
- Infusions—made in a similar way to tea, by steeping 2 teaspoons of dried herb or up to 4 teaspoons of a fresh herb in boiling water for 10 minutes. Strain, and add honey or sugar if necessary
- Ointments or creams applied topically
- Decoctions—the herbs and plant materials are boiled with water and reduced to made a thick soupy brew
- Suppositories or enemas
- Poultices
- Herbal baths
- Essences—a mixture of herbal essences which you burn and then inhale

Specific remedies

A number of plants have been found to be beneficial for specific conditions. You may find some of the following herbs valuable:
- St. John's wort (*Hypericum perforatum*) has undergone many scientific studies which show that it can lift mild depression.
- Garlic is used by herbalists to treat high blood pressure, arthritis, and asthma. About 30 scientific studies show that one clove of garlic a day (or the equivalent in a tablet) lowers cholesterol by 10–15 percent. Because it acts as an antibiotic, garlic is good for colds, coughs, sinusitis, and digestive disorders.
- Peppermint contains menthol, which relaxes the gut muscle. It is used to treat irritable bowel syndrome.
- *Echinacea purpurea* stimulates the immune system and boosts resistance to colds and viral infections.

Prepare a decoction by adding the fresh or dried herbs to water and boiling to reduce the liquid. Strain off the liquid and discard the solid matter.

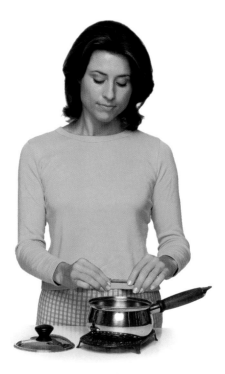
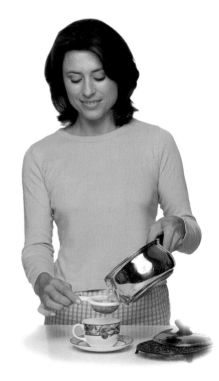

• Aloe vera is prescribed by herbalists for irritable bowel syndrome.

• Chamomile soothes an upset stomach, helps the digestion, and is a mild sedative.

• Valerian reduces tension and anxiety.

• Maitake mushrooms (*Grifola frondosa*), now marketed as pills, are said to boost the immune system.

Eczema

• Marigold (*Calendula officianalis*) is one of the best herbal remedies for eczema, burns, and bruises. Add 2 cups (500 ml) of boiling water to 1 oz (28 g) of marigold petals and leave to soak for 5 minutes. Strain and drink. You can also buy calendula cream.

• Chickweed can also be used for eczema and other itchy skin conditions.

Allergies

• Wild thyme is a powerful antibacterial agent. It is recommended by herbalists for allergies, digestive upsets, and arthritis.

• Hyssop is believed to be beneficial for hay fever and asthma, as well as colds, coughs, and congestion. Do not take hyssop during pregnancy.

• Nettle, taken in an infusion, can help soothe some allergic reactions.

• Marsh mallow and slippery elm soothe the gut and may ease the symptoms of celiac disease. Anti-inflammatory agents such as chamomile and meadowsweet may also help.

• Chickweed or chamomile, made into a cool infusion, can help relieve the itching of hives.

Asthma

An infusion of euphorbia mixed with thyme may help relax lung spasms and loosen phlegm.

Find out more

Chinese herbal medicine   112
Homeopathy   122

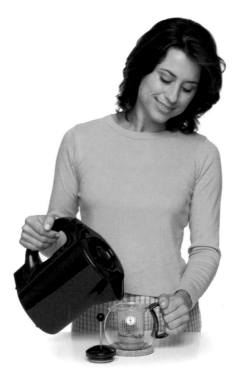

You can make an infusion as simply as brewing a cup of tea. Using a coffee maker with a plunger is a convenient way of separating the plant from the liquid.

WARNING

Not all herbs are good for you. Chaparral, promoted as a cancer and acne cure, comfrey root (but not the leaf), and coltsfoot have all been banned because they contain potentially toxic substances. Yohimbe, marketed as an aphrodisiac, and Ma huang, used for weight control, can be harmful. Ma huang, which comes from northern China, is the source of ephedrine, used in drugs for asthma, bronchitis, and emphysema. It should only be taken under supervision from a qualified herbal practitioner or doctor.

• Buy off-the-shelf herbal remedies from trusted and reputable outlets, such as drugstores and pharmacies, health food outlets, and supermarkets. Some pills and tablets may be contaminated with pesticides, fertilizers, and heavy metals, such as lead or mercury.

• Never collect herbs in the wild.

• If you are pregnant or breastfeeding and want to take an herbal remedy, ask your doctor or pharmacist if this is a good idea. Certain herbal remedies should not be used during pregnancy.

• If you are allergic to bee venom, you may have an allergic reaction to royal jelly capsules. If you are allergic to shellfish, anything with green-lipped mussels in it could trigger a reaction.

CHAPTER FOUR

Ayurvedic medicine

Practiced mainly in the Indian subcontinent, Ayurveda is an ancient holistic system of medicine. It is a blend of meditation, yoga, astrology, herbal medicine, massage, and dietary advice that encourages physical, emotional, spiritual, and mental health.

Diet is an important element in Ayurvedic medicine. A practitioner will recommend foods that are most suited to your dosha and will correct any constitutional imbalances.

The word "Ayurveda" comes from two Sanskrit words: *ayur*, or life, and *veda,* or knowledge, so Ayurveda means "the science of life." It was first described in the earliest Vedic texts, written by Hindu holy men, which date from around 2,500 BCE, but Ayurveda is believed to date back to more than 5,000 BCE, making it the most ancient of all medicinal systems. Ayurveda is little known outside Asia and Asian communities, but is just as comprehensive as, and similar to, Traditional Chinese Medicine.

It is practiced widely in Sri Lanka and India—there are 400,000 Ayurveda practitioners in India alone—and doctors in parts of Asia use Ayurveda alongside Western medicine and homeopathy.

In the West and particularly the U.S., it is mainly practiced in Maharishi Ayur-Ved centers, set up by followers of the Maharishi Mahesh Yogi, who founded the Transcendental Meditation movement. However, in countries with a sizable Asian immigrant population, such as the United Kingdom, there are numerous well-established networks of practitioners who have been trained in Asia.

The doshas

Ayurvedic practitioners believe that all living things comprise five elements—fire, water, earth, air, and ether—which are converted by *agni*, the digestive fire, into three humors, the *doshas*, or vital energies that influence both well-being and temperament.

The *doshas* are affected by diet, stress, and times of the day or year. Imbalances are thought to impede the flow of both *agni* and *prana*, the breath of life, which enters the body through food and breathing. As well as these, the third primal force, *soma*, a manifestation of love and harmony, can also be disturbed. Herbs and special diets aim to restore equilibrium.

Made up of two of the five elements, the *doshas* are fluctuating centers of energy. Air and ether form *vata; pitta* is produced from fire and water; and *kapha* is formed from water and earth. These *doshas* are fed by food, drink, fresh air, exercise, and spiritual activity. *Vata, pitta,* and *kapha* activity are said to be at their strongest at dawn, noon, and in the evening, respectively.

Visiting a practitioner

Your first visit will last about an hour and the practitioner will ask you about your lifestyle, diet, relationships at work, and your family life. He will take your pulse the doshic way, at three points on each wrist, and will examine your eyes, tongue, and nails for signs of doshic imbalance and toxic waste. The practitioner will also look at your build and features and work out which doshic type you are.

If you are strong enough, your treatment may start with a detoxification regime, since the elimination of toxic waste from your body underlies Ayurvedic medicine. This is called *shodan* and may involve enemas, purgatives, laxatives, and nasal washing as well as a dietary regime and saunas.

You may also be given *marma* massage, a therapeutic massage with oils, or *marma* puncture. According to Ayurvedic philosophy, the body has 107 vital points, or *marmas*, thought to correspond to organs or functions. Stimulating these points, either by massaging them or inserting needles, like acupuncture, is believed to bring about health and well-being.

For a *marma* massage the practitioner will deeply press parts of the back, neck, legs, arms, and hands to unblock the *marmas*. If the *marmas* are clear then you will stay balanced and healthy.

Medical products are prepared from plants using bark, root, fruit, leaves, and sometimes seeds. Minerals, sea shells, animal substances, and metals are also used. A health problem associated with excess phlegm, such as congestion and water retention, for example, would typically be treated with warm, light, dry foods and with fasting and avoiding cold drinks, which would increase *kapha*.

Herbal remedies may include hot spices such as cinnamon or cayenne; bitters such as turmeric; pungent tonics such as saffron; and stimulating herbs such as myrrh—all of which are designed to clear excess water or phlegm. Taste is also important in Ayurveda.

The practitioner may also suggest *rasayana*, a rejuvenating regime of yoga, chanting, meditation, and sunbathing. You may be asked to visit the practitioner once every two weeks for the first few months, then once a month.

The benefits

Ayurveda is good for skin conditions such as eczema, acne, and psoriasis; stress-related conditions such as migraines and fatigue; and indigestion, irritable bowel syndrome, stomach ulcers, and general digestive complaints.

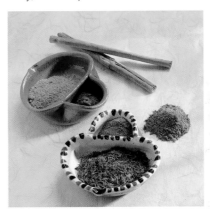

Bitter spices can reduce kapha, *so the diet may favor these over sweet, salty, or sour flavors.*

TYPE	CHARACTERISTICS	POTENTIAL PROBLEMS	FOOD TO AVOID	FOOD TO EAT
VATA	• Creative • Active • Restless	• Arthritis • Musculoskeletal problems • Irregular periods	Raw food	Moist, warming foods such as casseroles
PITTA	• Ambitious • Emotional • Intelligent	• Heartburn • Migraines • Allergies	Sour, salty, pungent foods such as red meat	Sweet, astringent, cold foods such as chicken, fish, salads, and tofu
KAPHA	• Happy • Peaceful	• Colds • Poor appetite • Allergies	Sweet, juicy vegetables	• Hot, spicy foods • Apples and pears • Leafy vegetables • Beans

Homeopathy

*T*he word "homeopathy" comes from the Greek homoios, *"like," and* pathos, *"suffering," and the principle underlying homeopathy is "like is cured by like." In other words, substances that cause certain symptoms in healthy people can cure sick people who are experiencing those symptoms.*

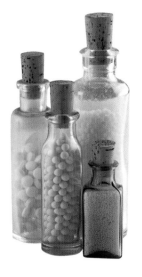

A homeopath may prescribe you a single remedy or several remedies combined into one pill.

Dr. Samuel Hahnemann, a German physician, established the principles of homeopathy in the late 18th century and is regarded as the father of homeopathy. Hahnemann devoted his life to testing a huge number of animal, vegetable, and mineral substances. He recruited healthy volunteers on whom he could test these substances before he tried them out on the sick and between 1790 and 1805 he tested 60 remedies.

Homeopathy is very different from orthodox medicine, which tries to suppress symptoms. If you have trouble sleeping, for example, a doctor will prescribe tablets that will bring on sleep artificially. A homeopath, however, will do exactly the opposite and prescribe minute quantities of a substance, such as coffee, which in large doses would almost certainly keep you awake. If you have hay fever, you may be prescribed a remedy made from a range of pollens.

The reactions of healthy volunteers, a process known as proving, have been documented in homeopathic handbooks, the most well known of which is Hahnemann's *Homeopathic Materia Medica* (1811).

Homeopathic dilution

The remedies are made from plants and minerals that are roughly chopped and left to soak in alcohol and water for several weeks and then sieved to form a "mother tincture." This is then diluted. It can either be diluted on the decimal or x scale, which has a dilution factor of 1:10, or on the centesimal, or c scale, with a dilution factor of 1:100. Between each dilution it is shaken rapidly, a process called "succussion." This is because

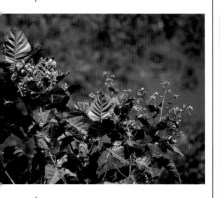

Many homeopathic remedies are based on plants, such as Cinchona.

CONSTITUTIONAL TYPES

Your constitutional type remains fixed throughout your life. Different types of people are categorized by the remedy that works best for them. There are many different types, but some of the most common are:
* Nux vomica *types are impatient, oversensitive and highly strung, with inner anger that may be repressed. They are likely to suffer from stress-related conditions such as insomnia, heartburn, irritable bowel syndrome and indigestion.*
* Pulsatilla *types are gentle, emotional and loving, but are prone to infections. If women, they often have menstrual problems.*
* Merc. sol *types are quick-tempered introverts, susceptible to respiratory conditions.*
* Apis *types are restless, unpredictable and moody. They often have outbursts of anger. They are prone to rashes and have hot, dry, sensitive skin.*

Hahnemann discovered that if he shook the remedy vigorously it seemed to increase its potency. Similarly, the more dilute the remedy the stronger and more effective it became. Dilutions of one part in a billion still appeared to work.

The process of diluting a remedy is known as potentization. Potentization means that poisons such as belladonna, arsenic, and strychnine (from *Nux vomica*), which would normally be poisonous, can safely be used.

Visiting a practitioner

Like all complementary therapies, homeopathy is a holistic system and is used to treat the whole person, not just the illness. While a conventional doctor will only diagnose and treat specific symptoms that point to a particular disease, homeopaths can treat ailments before they become apparent, when all you may feel is fatigue, or being under the weather—what homeopaths call "dis-ease."

Practitioners are either doctors who have been trained in homeopathic techniques or homeopaths who are not medically qualified. They may also be either "classical" or "complex" homeopaths.

A classical homeopath will use a single dose of the remedy that matches your constitutional type (see box). This takes enormous skill and you may have to visit the practitioner several times before you are prescribed the right remedy.

Complex practitioners look at the organic causes of the symptoms rather than the personality or what constitutional type you are. By matching remedies to specific individual symptoms, homeopaths claim to manipulate these energy patterns to bring about health.

Homeopathic remedies can come from an animal, such as snake venom (*Lachesis*), honeybee (*Apis*), or oyster shells (*Calcarea carbonica*); a plant, such as foxglove (*Digitalis*); or a mineral, such as silver nitrate (*Argent nit*) or sodium chloride (*Nat mur*). The skill of the practitioner is to find the exact remedy for your symptoms.

The remedies are prescribed as tablets, tinctures, powders, or granules, which should be taken between meals. You should not eat or drink anything for 20 minutes before and after taking the remedy. Most homeopaths suggest treating yourself with the 6th potency, roughly equivalent to a pinch of salt in a bath.

Homeopaths make a distinction between acute illnesses and chronic ailments, such as asthma and eczema. Long-term illnesses are seen as "constitutional" problems and you will probably be given a single remedy. Your homeopath will advise you to avoid coffee, cigarettes, peppermint, and preparations containing menthol, eucalyptus, and camphor because these can block the action of the remedy. You should store your remedies in a cool, dark place.

You may feel better almost immediately, or it may take months to recover from your illness. Some people find their symptoms initially get worse. You may develop a rash or cold or some kind of discharge. This is called the "initial aggravation" and is a sign that the medicine is working.

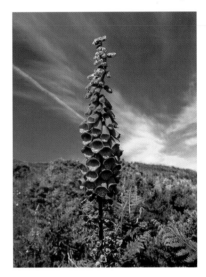

Foxglove is the source of the drug digitalis, used in modern medicine as a heart stimulant.

There are more than 3,000 remedies from which a homeopath can choose.

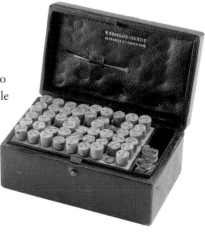

Osteopathy and chiropractic

Duuring the late 19th century osteopathy and chiropractic evolved in North America. Their main strengths lie in dealing with backache, neck pain, and other musculoskeletal disorders. They are now increasingly accepted by conventional medicine.

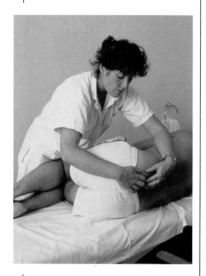

Osteopathy aims to treat illness by manipulation of the joints and muscles.

When it comes to treating asthma and allergies, osteopathy and chiropractic work by alleviating stress and tension, balancing or realigning the spine, and loosening the muscles which, in turn, will improve lung functions.

Both osteopathy and chiropractic are highly respected professions and in most countries practitioners are state-registered just like any other health professional. They practice alongside conventional medicine in North America, Australasia, and Europe.

Chiropractic

Practitioners believe that abnormalities in the joints and muscles are brought about through stress, poor posture, and accidents. They use their hands to manipulate joints and muscles in order to relieve pain and improve mobility. The word "chiropractic" comes from the Greek, *cheiro*, or hands, and *praktikos*, meaning "practice."

Chiropractic was developed by Daniel David Palmer, a Canadian grocer and "bonesetter" in 1895. He tested his theories on his office janitor, who had been deaf for 17 years following a back injury. Palmer examined his back and found a dislocated vertebra, which he manipulated, causing the janitor's hearing—unexpectedly—to return.

The theory behind the technique Palmer developed is that minor spinal displacements can cause nerve irritation, which in turn leads to disturbances of the nervous system and eventually illness. Chiropractors believe that many ailments begin in the spine. If the vertebrae are misaligned or maladjusted (what chiropractors refer to as "subluxed"), this not only restricts the nerves, causing pain, but also interferes with the body's "innate intelligence" or vital force.

Practitioners maintain that by adjusting these misaligned joints, or subluxations, chiropractic affects the nervous system. As a result, chiropractic can have a very positive effect on conditions that are not musculoskeletal in origin, such as asthma and irritable bowel syndrome.

Palmer set up the Palmer Infirmary and Chiropractic Institute in Iowa, and the profession grew rapidly, spreading across the U.S. and onto Australia, New Zealand, and Europe.

GENTLER VARIETIES

Two English chiropractors, John McTimoney and Hugh Corley, developed two variations of standard chiropractic called McTimoney and McTimoney–Corley chiropractic.

McTimoney chiropractic was developed in the 1950s and practitioners say their adjustment techniques are gentler, with fewer high-velocity thrusts, so it is suitable for the elderly as well as for people who dislike the thrusts of standard chiropractic.

McTimoney therapists use a manipulation called toggle recoil, which "springs" the joints. They say the technique is very fast and you hardly feel a thing. McTimoney chiropractors also treat musculoskeletal problems in horses, cats, dogs, and farm animals. Corley trained under McTimoney and developed his own gentle technique, in which only fingertips are used to manipulate and adjust.

Visiting a practitioner

The osteopath or chiropractor will begin by taking a medical history, which will include any accidents—even minor ones—you may have had in the past. He or she will ask you about your lifestyle and observe your posture and the way you walk, and ask you to undress to your underwear to see how your muscles and spine work.

The practitioner will palpate your spine, pressing each vertebra in turn and finding out which one is painful. He or she will probably ask you to slide your arms down your sides, raise your legs, and ask you to bend over, to see if this hurts your spine. A chiropractor may also take X rays, check your blood pressure, and test your reflexes.

Chiropractors usually have special tables so that they can position you for manipulation and to minimize any pain in lying down and standing up. They use around 150 techniques, working on the skin, muscles, and connective tissue to stretch and relax the muscles. They also use high-velocity thrusts to adjust joints, particularly in the neck and lower back and this may be used two or three times in a session.

The high-velocity thrusts are not at all painful, but you will hear an unnerving cracking sound, similar to fingers cracking. This is caused by gas bubbles in the fluid surrounding the joints bursting under pressure. The thrust is short and precise and requires a great deal of expertise on the part of the chiropractor. Many people say that they feel considerably "freed up" and revitalized after treatment.

Chiropractic is mainly used to treat neck, shoulder, back, and arm pain, along with headaches and migraines due to tension, joint problems, sports injuries to the knee, ankle, hands, and feet. Only on occasion do chiropractors treat diseases with an organic nature, such as asthma, irritable bowel syndrome, some types of migraines and headaches, and painful menstruation. This is not to say that asthma, for instance, does not respond well to manipulative treatment—anything that frees the chest and encourages good posture will help asthma symptoms. ▶

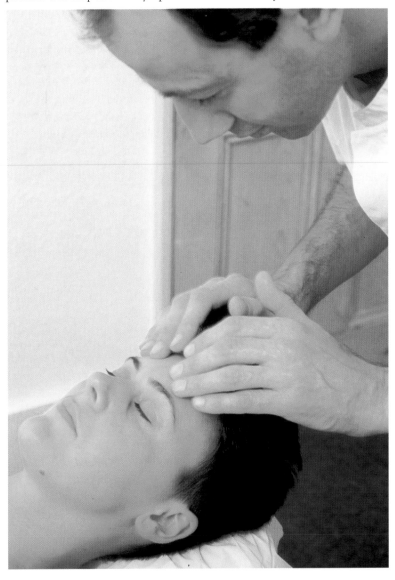

Manipulation of the neck and head is a common part of a treatment by a chiropractor.

CHAPTER FOUR

Osteopathy and chiropractic

Osteopathy

The word "osteopathy" comes from two Greek words: *osteo* (bone) and *pathos* (disease). As in chiropractic, the practitioner manipulates and adjusts the bones, joints, muscles, ligaments, and connective tissue to bring about well-being.

Osteopaths believe that what they refer to as osteopathic lesions are imbalances in the normal tension of the spine. Through their effect on the nervous system, these lesions may be the origin of discomfort or malfunction elsewhere in the body.

Working with their hands, osteopaths treat all parts of the body, including the back, head, wrists, shoulders, elbows, knees, ankles, and feet. Osteopathy is in many ways similar to chiropractic, but

Osteopaths apply the same principles to children as to adults, but the treatment is usually much gentler.

osteopaths concentrate more on soft tissue techniques to relax the muscles. Another difference is that chiropractors make extensive use of X rays in order to diagnose problems, while osteopaths rely on their knowledge of the human body to ascertain where there is dysfunction and immobility.

An American doctor and engineer, Andrew Taylor Still, founded osteopathy in 1874. He was devastated by the loss of his wife and three of his children in a meningitis epidemic and could not understand why doctors had failed to save them. Spurred on by the tragedy, he began to examine the body and became convinced that it could not function properly unless it was structurally sound.

Still was a deeply religious man and believed that the body was created by God in His own image and once restored to its original design would be able to

PEDIATRIC OSTEOPATHY

Many childhood ailments, practitioners say, can be traced back to unresolved strains experienced during birth, which can lead to nervous disorders and behavioral problems. Babies have a drive toward the "normal," so the sooner the osteopath gets his or her hands on a baby the better. Osteopaths aim to rebalance the body to enable the child to harness his or her own vital forces.

Practitioners treat all parts of the body, not just the head, but when an osteopath treats babies and children the touch is light and they rarely use the crunching, high-velocity thrust used on adults.

heal itself. By osteopathic readjustment, the body's natural healing life-force would restore it to health.

The thinking behind his treatment was that where blood circulated normally, disease could not develop. Once it became sluggish, however, it would go "sour" and disease would follow. Still not only treated musculoskeletal problems but also tackled tuberculosis, gallstones, epilepsy, and tumors. In 1892, he set up a school of osteopathy in Kirksville, Missouri, and wrote down his techniques in *The Osteopathic Blue Book*.

Visiting a practitioner

Many aspects of treatment by an osteopath and a chiropractor are similar. A number of the diagnostic techniques that they use are the same—testing your blood pressure and reflexes, taking X rays, and observing your posture.

However, an osteopath will pay close attention to your body to make sure that it is symmetrical. He or she will look at the length of your legs to see if they are the same and examine your hips to see if they tilt to one side or not. You will be asked to lie on a table and much of the session will be taken up with work on the skin, muscles, and connective tissue of your body, with you lying on your side, back, or front.

Techniques employed by an osteopath include massage to relax stiff muscles, stretching to help joint mobility, and manipulation or high-velocity thrusting, which restores easy movement to the body. Sometimes the practitioner will use indirect techniques, which involve light touching and gentle positioning of the joints to reduce tension and restore balance.

One session may be enough to restore you to health, but if you have a chronic problem then you will almost certainly be advised to have more. Three to six sessions are average and many people benefit from going for a replenishment session every few months.

Who can benefit?

Osteopathy is mainly used to treat a variety of musculoskeletal problems, and half the workload of osteopaths consists of helping people with back pain. The therapy has had great success in treating both chronic and acute back pain. However, osteopaths say that the techniques can also relieve conditions such as bronchitis, constipation, and premenstrual tension. Osteopathy is also used to strengthen the immune system. If you have asthma, osteopaths can help you by using manipulation to open the chest, stretch the diaphragm, and improve posture.

Cranial osteopathy

A separate, but related, discipline, known as cranial osteopathy, was developed in the 1950s by William Garner Sutherland. Sutherland, an American osteopath, studied under Andrew Still. He became particularly interested in the bones of the skull, which are separate in babies but become fixed in adults. Sutherland found that these bones were still capable of some movement in adults and that pressing these bones could produce strong physical and emotional reactions.

Sutherland developed a theory that states that cerebrospinal fluid flows in rhythmic pulses. By gentle manipulation of the skull, cranial osteopathy can discover any irregularities in these pulses and restore the flow to its natural rhythm.

The Alexander technique

*T**he Alexander technique is similar to yoga, t'ai chi, and qigong in as much as you need a practitioner to teach you; but once learned you can incorporate it into your daily life.***

The Alexander technique was invented by an Australian actor, Frederick Matthias Alexander. He was born in 1869 in Tasmania. The stress of performing affected his voice. Often he could barely finish a recitation. Doctors advised him to "rest" his voice, but this had little or no effect and hardly helped his career.

Alexander devised a technique that cured his voice. In addition, he found that the postural techniques also seemed to cure his bad temper and he became a more positive and likeable personality.

He came to the conclusion that the head, neck, and spine were interconnected and what we did with one affected the others and the health of all the organs.

The importance of posture

Most adults have terrible posture and many of these habits were picked up in childhood. Children get plenty of education about brushing their teeth and making sure their shoes fit, but the spine is rather neglected.

Poor posture not only leads to wear and tear on the lower lumbar region of the back and base of the neck, it weakens the back muscles, puts pressure on joints and ligaments, and stores up trouble for

later life. By preventing full abdominal breathing, bad posture constricts blood vessels, starving the organs of oxygen and nutrients, and compresses the stomach and lungs leading to poor digestion, asthma, and a host of other conditions.

Visiting an Alexander teacher

Wear something loose, like leggings or a tracksuit. The teacher will observe you walking around the room and sitting down to see how you use your body. You will be asked whether you are active in your work or whether you spend a lot of time behind a desk, and whether you have had any accidents in the past.

Once the teacher has observed you, you will lie on a couch, with your head on a small pile of two or three books and your knees raised. The teacher will use his or her hands to persuade or "direct" your limbs to adopt correct positions.

It is a gentle method—teachers simply lay their hands on various parts of the body. They may ask you to "give" them the full weight of your arm. The more tense you are, the harder it is to do this.

Sometimes the teacher will ask you to "think" through various muscles. You will be asked to concentrate on your muscles and "think" that the ankles and heels are rooted to the floor, or that there is an eye on the top of your head looking toward the sky and lifting your spine up.

The teacher will draw your attention to your posture, and explain the best way to achieve a more natural posture. You may find you have "grown" by an inch or so after the lesson.

Lie down on the floor with a couple of books under your head and the knees bent upward for about 20 minutes. Make sure your spine is flat and "think" your lower lumbar region into the floor. Keep your chin in and breathe naturally. This exercise will correct any exaggerated curve of the neck and will straighten the spine.

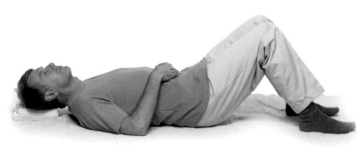

ALEXANDER PRINCIPLES

Alexander teachers believe that ill health comes from poor "use of self." Proper "use," what Alexander called "primary control," comes from being aware of how you sit, stand, and move.

Most people slump when they stand up, with rounded shoulders, a caved-in chest, a slack stomach, and knees that are slightly bent. The pelvis may jut out in front of the body. Asked to stand straight, they thrust out the chest, curve the back, and stiffen the neck and legs.

Good posture, or primary control as taught by Alexander teachers, involves lengthening the spine and pulling it up, as if you have a thread through your skull that pulls you toward the sky.

Your shoulders and neck should be relaxed, your head pulled slightly back, your torso should widen out, and your spine should be straight but never arched. This opening of the body reduces pressure on the heart, lungs, stomach, intestines, and other organs.

Alexander technique is good for stress-related conditions such as anxiety and hypertension. Most people do something as quickly as possible without giving it a thought (Alexander called this "endgain"). They sit and stand up quickly, do several things at one time, bolt down food, and use an unnecessary amount of energy, in all kinds of ways, just doing daily tasks.

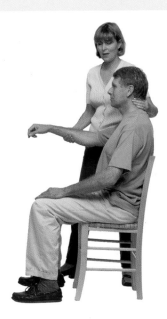
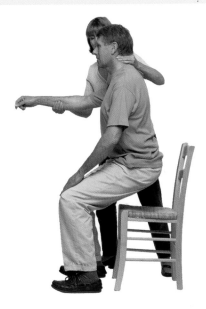
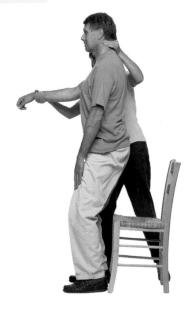

1 To get out of a chair, start by sitting near the front of the chair and place your hands on your lap. Keep your hands apart.

2 Curve your head forward and upward as you lean forward from the hips. Your weight is now transferred to your feet.

3 Keeping your back straight and directing your head forward and upward, keep your knees apart as you straighten your legs.

Nutritional therapy

All complementary therapies emphasize the need for a healthy diet full of fresh vegetables, fruit, and whole grains. Nutritional therapy works on the basis of recommending particular nutrients, such as vitamins, minerals, or amino acids, to cure an ailment.

Research shows that a plentiful intake of fresh fruit and vegetables—at least five portions a day—builds up resistance to disease and may guard against cancer, coronary heart disease, and cataracts. Nutritional therapy, or nutritional medicine, aims to treat disease with particular vitamins, minerals, amino acids, and other nutrients, often in supplement form. This is different from naturopathy, where the emphasis is on wholefoods, exercise, and hydrotherapy.

Nutritional therapists believe that the modern diet, however balanced you believe it to be, is lacking in essential nutrients and that what constitutes a healthy diet for one person may not be adequate for another. Illness, practitioners believe, is caused by biochemical abnormalities and an alteration in the normal processing of nutrients. By correcting these with nutritional supplements, symptoms can be alleviated.

A poor diet, high in saturated fats and low in fiber, has been linked to cancer of the rectum, breast, and prostate, while a diet high in fruit and vegetables has been shown to protect against coronary heart disease. A diet high in salt makes your airways react more strongly to histamine, and alcohol restricts the bronchi.

The magic ingredients in fruit and vegetables are antioxidants—vitamins C, E, and A (betacarotene), and minerals— which the body uses as its frontline troops against chemicals called free radicals, by-products of the body's metabolism.

Body cells are made up of molecules, and most molecules have an even number of electrons, which makes them stable. But the free radicals have an extra electron each and race around the body looking for a mate, either to steal an electron from or to donate the spare electron to.

The free radicals' job is to turn food and oxygen into energy, and in a healthy body they normally disappear within microseconds. But when you have too many of them, either through age, illness, or external sources such as cigarette smoke or pollution, they can slowly destroy the body, snatching away electrons from healthy cells. Their scavenging activities are now believed to trigger cancer and heart disease and cause damage to the immune system.

The body deals with free radicals with its army of antioxidants. These, too, have spare electrons, which they donate to cells that have been attacked by free radicals. Antioxidants are the key to good health and the better your diet, the healthier you are, and the more efficient this fighting system will be. Studies have shown that

Juices of fruit and vegetables are delicious and easy to prepare. They are an excellent source of vitamins and minerals.

doses of vitamin E and betacarotene could cut deaths from prostate cancer by 34 percent, stomach cancer by 21 percent, and cancer overall by 13 percent. An antioxidant-rich diet can help keep your heart healthy, reduce strokes, and prolong life in the elderly.

Antioxidants

The main sources of antioxidants are the following:
• Vitamin A (betacarotene): carrots, spinach, broccoli, tomatoes.
• Vitamin C: citrus fruits, kiwi fruit, peas, potatoes, green leafy vegetables.
• Vitamin E: wheat germ, nuts, green leafy vegetables, whole-wheat bread, vegetable oils, particularly sunflower and rapeseed, spinach, and avocado.
• Minerals: selenium, zinc, copper, niacin, vitamin B_1 and B_{12}, folic acid, pantothenic acid, magnesium, and manganese—all found in fruit and vegetables, plus organ meats, wheat germ, whole-wheat bread, oily fish, and dairy products.

Visiting a practitioner

You may be asked to complete a questionnaire about your health and diet, how much you drink and smoke, your lifestyle, and any medication you are taking. The practitioner will look at your skin, eyes, and nails, and question you about your mood and stress levels.

You may be diagnosed through hair, urine, or blood tests, a Vega machine, or applied kinesiology. You will be asked to exclude tea, coffee, alcohol, chocolate, salt, salted foods, red meat, sugar, and saturated fats from your diet. You may be placed on an elimination diet to pinpoint any food allergies.

Using information gained through the diagnosis, the practitioner will devise a treatment tailored to your needs. He or she may recommend a diet rich in a particular nutrient, which may be supplemented with doses of that nutrient in the form of capsules, powders, or liquids. In some cases nutritional therapists give injections of supplements.

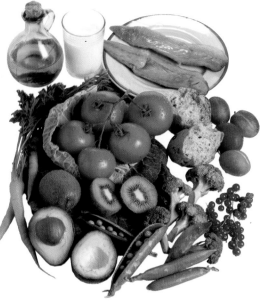

Fresh fruit and vegetables, whole-wheat bread, vegetable oils, and oily fish are all sources of antioxidants, now considered an important part of a healthy diet.

WARNING

• *It is wise to visit your doctor before starting on a regime of vitamin and mineral supplementation. Excessive doses of vitamins A, D, E, B_6, and zinc can be harmful.*
• *Don't put your child on a low-fat, sugar-free diet. An adult low-fat, high-fiber, low-meat diet is not right for children, particularly those under two, and may stunt their physical and mental development. Babies and toddlers need whole milk and sugary foods, and have a natural sweet tooth—instinctively they know what is good for them. Neither sugar nor fat makes a child obese—overeating does.*

Nutritional therapy

Staying healthy

• Eat a low-allergy diet, avoiding common food allergens, such as cow's milk, oranges, eggs, and, if you feel you have a sensitivity, wheat products.

• Keep your baby healthy by breastfeeding for as long as possible and avoiding foods with nuts in them. Keep your intake of peanuts to a minimum when breastfeeding.

• Serve fruit and vegetables raw where possible. Or, steam or stir-fry them and leave the skins on.

• If you are on medication, take an antioxidant supplement. Drugs speed up the activity of the liver, which means that it works overtime, eliminating not only the drug but healthy nutrients too.

• Avoid fad foods and diets; very often they contain little more than preservatives and empty calories. Your health will suffer if these become the basis of your diet.

• Reintroduce foods slowly into your diet; citrus fruits in particular need to be reintroduced one at a time.

Supplements that may help with your asthma and allergies

• Magnesium: several studies have shown that wheezing is related to low levels of magnesium in the blood.

• Selenium: research shows that asthma is linked to reduced levels of this antioxidant mineral. In one study, people who suffered from asthma were given selenium supplements and showed considerable improvement.

• Vitamin B_6: supplements have been shown to alleviate asthma symptoms.

• Vitamin B_{12}: supplements can reduce asthma symptoms. In one study of 85 asthma patients, all benefited from 1,000 mcg of vitamin B_{12} injected once a week—the younger the patient, the better the response to the treatment.

• Vitamin C: high-dose supplements can reduce asthma attacks. In one study of children, those who had 1 gram of vitamin C a day for two weeks had one-quarter fewer attacks than those who had been given a dummy treatment.

• Essential fatty acids: studies show that omega-3 essential fatty acids, contained in fish oils, improve asthma symptoms.

Whether you follow a nutritionist's advice or create your own eating plan, take a multivitamin and mineral supplement every day to ensure you get the nutrients that your body needs.

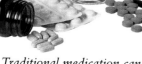

Traditional medication can speed up the activity in your liver. Take an antioxidant to counteract any negative effects.

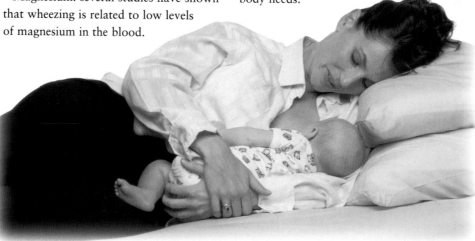

Be careful with your diet when breastfeeding your baby. Avoid nuts in particular; they are a known source of allergens.

Naturopathy

"*Nature cure," or naturopathy, treats body and mind together. It is a multidisciplinary therapy that uses diet, exercise, spinal manipulation, herbs, massage, and hydrotherapy to restore you to a point at which your body will heal itself.*

Find out more

Food allergies	72
Herbal medicine	116
Massage	138

An unhealthy diet, stress, a polluted environment, lack of sleep, and an unhappy home or work life encourage toxins to built up in the body, damaging the body's inner vitality and allowing disease to thrive. Practitioners of naturopathy do not treat symptoms because, like most complementary therapists, they see symptoms as a manifestation of the body's healing forces, or defenses, at work, and maintain that these should not be suppressed. If they are treated and suppressed, the disease may become chronic and cause further damage and degeneration in the body.

A natural lifestyle is at the heart of naturopathy and its fundamental principles are that the secret to a long healthy life is eating plain wholesome food, getting fresh air and plenty of exercise, and keeping a positive outlook.

Naturopaths talk of the "triad of health"—biochemical, structural, and psychological. So practitioners will treat your biochemical imbalances with fasting, adjustments in diet, and herbal remedies. Your structural misalignment will be treated with massages, postural exercises to develop your flexibility, and osteopathic or chiropractic manipulation and massage. Your mental health will be improved through better nutrition and counseling.

Hydrotherapy uses water to heal in the form of hot and cold showers, special baths, and body wraps to stimulate circulation, reduce inflammation, and relieve congestion in the body leading to increased health and well-being.

Naturopaths will treat most illnesses, but often see people with chronic conditions such as migraine, fatigue, eating disorders, respiratory problems such as asthma and hay fever, skin problems, and arthritis. Asthma has developed differently in many parts of the world, so treatments can be diverse. In Europe, practitioners use more hydrotherapy and herbal agents; in the United States naturopaths specialize in herbal or homeopathic treatments and rely on blood and urine tests. In the United Kingdom, the emphasis is on fasting and dietary therapy.

The Greek physician Hippocrates was one of the first people to realize the importance of nature's own healing powers. In the guidelines he laid down for good health, he advocated rest, plain food, and plenty of exercise.

Health exponents of the naturopathic diet were the American Dr. Henry Lindlahr and the Swiss Dr. Max Bircher-Benner, the creator of muesli. Dr. Lindlahr, who laid down the ground rules for naturopathy, described the "accumulation of waste matter, morbid materials, and poisons" and said that their management required an adequate amount of fruit, vegetables, and whole grains—foods now widely recognized as protecting against cancer and other degenerative diseases.

Making a note of your symptoms and what seems to trigger them will help your practitioner to diagnose your problems.

Naturopathy

Some naturopaths use a technique called hair mineral analysis. A sample of hair is processed in a laboratory to test for any imbalances, which may then be corrected by an appropriate diet.

Visiting a practitioner

Naturopaths undergo similar training to that of a conventional doctor and use the same basic diagnostic techniques. They have two aims: first, to assist you in self-healing and, second, to introduce you to a healthier lifestyle for the long-term. During the first session, which can last up to an hour, the practitioner will ask a series of questions, which allows him or her to build up a detailed picture of your lifestyle and personal background as well as a medical history. He or she will also take your blood pressure and pulse, look at your posture, and ask you about your diet. The practitioner also needs to know whether you are stressed, what makes you happy, and whether or not you exercise. He or she will be particularly interested in any history of illness in your immediate family.

Once an idea of your lifestyle has been formed, the practitioner can begin to address your problem. When the underlying cause of your troubles has been diagnosed, the naturopath will draw up a plan for treatment, which varies according to the individual and their condition. Treatments are either anabolic—that is, they are designed to build you up—or catabolic, which means they cleanse you and break down the toxins that have accumulated in your body.

Naturopaths believe that toxicity is a major cause of illness and that there is a strong connection between toxins and allergies. For this reason, the most common treatments will include changes to your diet—practitioners believe that this can cure 8 out of 10 people. They normally recommend a diet that is biologically aligned, which means plenty of fresh fruit and vegetables—preferably organic—freshly squeezed mixed vegetable and fruit juices, no sugar or refined foods, a small amount of free-range meat, and no tobacco, alcohol, tea, or coffee. In addition, you may be put on an exclusion diet in order to discover the foods to which you have an intolerance.

In some instances, a total detoxification may be recommended to rid your body of poison. This may take the form of a short fast lasting between three and five days. At its strictest, you are only allowed to drink distilled water during the fast, although some fruit or vegetable juices may be permitted. You should rest during this period, avoiding all stressful activity and the use of chemicals such as soaps and skin lotions.

Practitioners believe that dairy products and sugar disturb the biochemistry of the body, making it more susceptible to bronchial spasm, and often suggest that you remove them from your diet. Hydrotherapy treatments such as hot and cold baths or compresses are sometimes recommended to stimulate the removal of toxins from your body. If you have a bronchial condition, you may be advised to apply hot and cold compresses to your chest, throat, or abdomen.

WARNING

Any fast or special diet should always be closely monitored. Children need fat, sugars, and carbohydrates, and should not be put on a low-fat diet.

You may experience what naturopaths call healing crisis after a few weeks. You may have loose bowels, a rash, or a fever, and if you have bronchitis, you may develop a chesty cough. This is regarded as a sign that the treatment is working and is sometimes enhanced by fever therapy, in which hydrotherapy or herbal medicines are used to elevate your body temperature and flush out the toxins. Keep in contact with your naturopath so that any changes or improvements in your symptoms can be monitored.

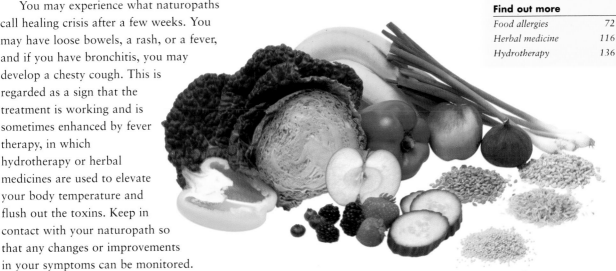

A NATUROPATHIC ANTIALLERGY REGIME

Include plenty of fresh fruit and vegetables in your diet and substitute legumes for red meat.

• *Eat plenty of fresh fruit and vegetables, but avoid citrus fruits, especially oranges and orange juice. Drink natural apple or grape juice, diluted with mineral water. Keep the skins on fruit and vegetables whenever possible.*

• *Reduce, and if possible cut out, your intake of all dairy products. This is particularly important if you suffer from asthma or eczema, because dairy products are known triggers of these complaints.*

• *If you do not want to give up meat completely, eat red meat once or twice a week at most. Compensate for the lack of meat by eating plenty of legumes.*

• *Get plenty of exercise. Do something physical at least two or three times a week—it will improve your circulation and strengthen your lungs.*

• *Do daily breathing exercises, remembering to keep your shoulders back to increase the volume of air that you can inhale.*

• *Cold showers will improve the circulation to areas affected by eczema. New scientific research has shown that taking a shower in the morning washes away dust mites and alleviates eczema.*

• *Use a loofah or body brush before a bath or shower to stimulate the circulation of your blood and eliminate toxins from your body.*

• *Avoid hot, stuffy, centrally heated atmospheres. Whenever possible, open a small window and use a humidifier to prevent the atmosphere from drying out.*

• *If you suffer from asthma, consider osteopathy: specific treatment to the thoracic region of the spine at the back of your chest can be beneficial.*

Hydrotherapy

*T*he treatment known as hydrotherapy consists of drinking or swimming in warm mineral water, inhaling its steam, having massages, as well as mud treatment, in which you are encased in clay that is "matured" and stiff with mineral salts and algae.

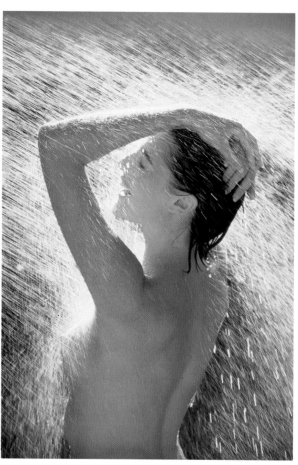

Taking a bracing cold shower first thing in the morning will stimulate your circulatory system.

Orthodox medicine now accepts hydrotherapy as a form of physiotherapy, but the healing properties of water have been recognized since ancient times. People have been bathing in the sea and "taking the waters" at spas for centuries, and it has long been accepted that hot and cold baths stimulate the circulation of the blood. Facilities included spinal washing, steam baths, abdominal compresses, head and foot baths, and other bracing regimes designed to tone up the nervous system, which in turn helped the body to overcome disease more effectively. Similar thinking still underpins hydrotherapy treatment today. Recent studies of hydrotherapy have shown that warm mineral water and mud have specific effects, which vary from spa to spa. It is believed that drinking particular mineral waters can cure a host of digestive disorders, while inhaling a steam solution distilled from certain mineral-rich waters is reputed to be good for respiratory problems. Sulfur waters are reputedly beneficial for asthma, bronchitis, and sinusitis, while plastering mud on the body is said to help circulatory problems, eczema and psoriasis.

The facilities of modern spas include warm thermal water—rich in sulfur, salts, iodine, and other minerals—mud baths, iodine-brine therapy, carbon dioxide baths, sulfur-water steam inhalations and mouth douches, whirlpool baths, Turkish baths, saunas, steam rooms, and bracing showers. There are a number of specialized treatments:

• Hot baths, used to loosen muscles, ease joint pain, and reduce inflammation. With the addition of seaweed or mineral salts, hot baths can be used as a mild antiseptic to heal minor grazes and cuts.

• Steam baths, Turkish baths, and saunas promote sweating, which opens the pores of your skin and cleanses your body of impurities. They are followed up with a dip in a cool plunge pool or bath.

• Fangotherapy, or mud treatment. The mud, which is also sometimes called curative bog, is enriched with thermal water, mineral salts, and algae, and then matured in vats before it is smoothed onto your body. It stimulates circulation, removes toxins, and soothes the skin.

• Thallasotherapy is a treatment involving seawater and seaweed (kelp), in which you either bathe or are encased. Seawater is believed to have healing properties that cleanse and tone the skin, induce sweating and promote relaxation.

• Sitz bathing involves placing two hip baths opposite each other—one containing cold water and the other hot.

You sit in the hot bath for 2–3 minutes and then in the cold bath for a minute, keeping your feet in the opposite bath.

• Compresses are small towels or cloths soaked in hot or cold mineral water, wrung out, and applied to a specific part of the body. Hot and cold compresses are alternated for maximum effect.

• Wraps are used to treat fever and backache. Cold sheeting is wrapped around your body, followed by a dry sheet, and finally a warm blanket. They are left in place until the inner sheet is dry, after which you sponge your body with tepid water and towel yourself dry.

• Flotation is a form of sensory deprivation involving lying face upward in a shallow, dark, enclosed tank of heavily salted warm water for a length of time. It is intended to be deeply relaxing and can induce an almost trancelike state in your mind or even a deep sleep.

There is biochemical evidence that when you immerse yourself in mineral water, there is a significant rise in the production of anti-inflammatory hormones known as endorphins, which ease pain. Researchers say that 88 percent of people with degenerative arthritis claim to have been helped by spa treatment.

Drinking spa water can ease an irritable bowel and help constipation. Breathing steaming spa water can clear the sinuses, and one study has found that when asthmatic children had spa therapy, the number of days they were forced to stay home from school through illness was substantially reduced. Studies have also shown that taking spa waters can stimulate bone cell growth in patients with osteoporosis and help treat skin ailments such as eczema and psoriasis by encouraging underlying cells to produce healthy new tissue.

Urine therapy

Western physicians do not recommend this, but urine therapy is well established in India. Urine is only water containing mineral salts, hormones, and the waste chemical urea, which is formed by the breakdown of nitrogen compounds and acts as an emollient, trapping water in the skin. Applied externally, urine is reputed to clear skin conditions such as eczema. In the past, bricklayers used to urinate on their hands to prevent dermatitis, and mothers used to wipe the faces of their babies with wet diapers to bring a bloom to their skin.

Home remedies

• Plunge your face into cold water first thing in the morning. This will stimulate your circulation and act as a decongestant.

• Immerse yourself in a hot bath for five minutes to relax tired muscles. The optimum temperature is between 98°F (36.5°C) and 104°F (40°C).

• Ease mild eczema by taking a tepid bath with 2 lb (1 kg) of salt dissolved in it. Remember, however, to avoid this if your skin is cracked and bleeding.

• Devise your own sitz bath using two basins or baby baths. A sitz bath may relieve such disorders as constipation.

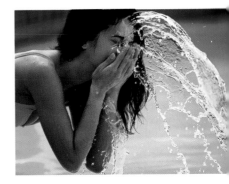

Splashing cold water onto your face refreshes your skin and can help to clear your nasal passages.

THE THERAPEUTIC FISH

The most unusual hydrotherapeutic treatment is found in India, where hundreds of thousands of asthmatics flock annually to Hyderabad to swallow a tiny fish called a murrel. The mouth of each 2-in (5-cm) long fish is stuffed with an herbal paste and then swallowed whole—and alive. On its way down into the stomach, the fish dislodges layers of phlegm and, once there, it releases the therapeutic herbs and dies. The recommended cure for asthma is to swallow one fish a year for three years.

Massage therapy

The word "massage" derives from the Greek massein—*"to knead"—and is a therapy based on the instinctive human need to touch and rub, either to comfort someone or to ease aches or pains in a specific part of the body. It is a holistic technique, combining the soothing qualities of touch with the manipulation of muscles, tendons, and ligaments.*

Manipulation is said to stimulate the blood and lymph flow, ease stiff muscles and joints, improve digestion, boost energy, and disperse accumulated toxins. There are many different types of massage, from traditional Swedish techniques to Thai massage to deep-tissue Indian *marma* massage. You can choose from manual lymph drainage, Indian head massage, touch therapies such as Reiki, or deep, sometimes painful, techniques such as Rolfing.

Massage is one of the oldest healing arts and most cultures throughout history have used it to heal and bring comfort. It is part of Ayurveda and Traditional Chinese Medicine, and before the advent of modern medicine it was used to cure everything from a bad back to chronic disease.

The Greeks and Romans used massage to prepare their gladiators for battle and Hippocrates prescribed it for his patients in 460 BC, stating that "the physician must be experienced in ... rubbing. For rubbing can bind a joint that is too loose and loosen a joint that is too rigid."

Various techniques were perfected by Middle Eastern and Asian cultures and are used regularly not only in their systems of medicine but in their daily lives. However, in the West, massage fell out of favor and was revived only in the 19th century by a Swedish gymnast, Per Henrik Ling. He developed his "Swedish movement technique," known as Swedish

massage, upon which most styles of European massage are based. His techniques were introduced into the United States around 1870.

During both World Wars, massages were used to rehabilitate injured soldiers, and were found to be particularly beneficial for those suffering from shell-shock. Massages became popular again in the 1970s, but developed a reputation, highly unjustifiably, for being sleazy. Swedish massage in particular became linked with sexual activities, so much so that reputable therapists now prefer to call themselves massage therapists or practitioners.

Today massage is used in many ways: by professionals wanting to relax after a hard week at the office; by people wanting to treat their aches and pains or just to pamper themselves, and by nurses and therapists in hospitals to treat the sick, the elderly, the terminally ill, and those in pain.

Swedish, or Western, massage is the most common form of massage and is often used in gyms and health clubs. Therapists usually use their hands and concentrate on easing tension in the muscles. Oils are often used to prevent friction, and aromatherapy oils can provide added benefits.

Oriental massage involves the therapist stimulating the acupressure points with his or her elbows and knees as well as hands and palms. Sometimes oils are used and the aim of the treatment is to release vitality and promote harmony in both mind and body. The four main forms of Oriental massage are Thai, shiatsu, Reiki, and tuina.

The University of Miami School of Medicine's Touch Institute has shown that massages have many benefits. They make people more alert, relieve anxiety and depression, increase the number of "killer" immune cells in the body, and lower the levels of the stress hormone called cortisol.

Scientists also found that premature babies whom they gently massaged three times a day for 15 minutes gained nearly 50 percent more weight and left the hospital six days earlier than babies who were not massaged. Many studies show that massage can help with childhood illnesses such as eczema, asthma, and diabetes, and it is a good way to help a child "wind down" after a busy day, thereby promoting sleep.

Other studies show that massage can help anxiety and depression and improve blood circulation, leading to a feeling of warmth and aiding the circulation of lymph around the body. A well-functioning lymphatic system acts as a drainage canal network, removing excess fluid from body tissues and returning it to the bloodstream. It also helps fight infection.

Treatment

At your first session, the therapist will ask you about your health, medical history, what medication you are taking, and your lifestyle. He or she will also want to know what sort of work you do and whether you have any particular stresses. Remember not to eat or drink immediately before a session.

If you have chosen a traditional massage, you can either have a full body massage or a neck and shoulder massage. For a full massage you will have to undress, but most people leave their underpants on. The therapist will use a towel to cover areas that are not currently being massaged.

Most therapists begin by treating the back first, followed by the neck and legs, sometimes using scented oils or, occasionally, talcum powder. Next the therapist will massage your shoulders, the front of your legs, arms, hands, and sometimes your abdomen. Most practitioners prefer to work in silence so they can concentrate on your body, but if you feel uncomfortable about anything or the massage hurts, voice your concerns. A massage should be enjoyable—not a cause of further stress.

A massage takes about an hour (30 minutes for neck and shoulders) and you will be left alone for a few minutes to rest at the end. You should feel warm and fully relaxed.

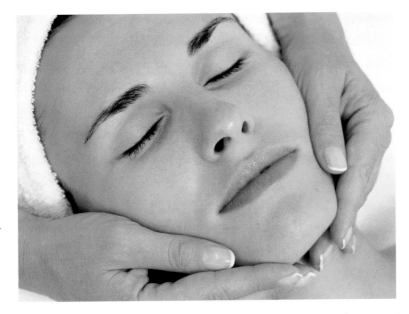

If you don't have time for a whole-body massage, a soothing facial massage can help to relieve tension.

Massage therapy

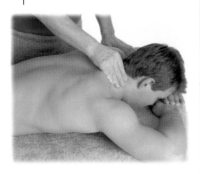

Massage benefits the neck muscles by improving circulation in the area and promoting relaxation.

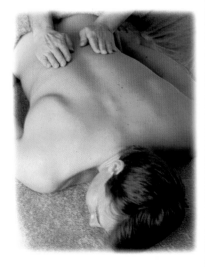

Apply even pressure so that the fingers exert the same pressure as the palm

THE BASIC STROKES

It is not difficult to learn basic massage strokes in order to give a massage.

Effleurage

Place some oil on your hands and glide them over long stretches of the body, such as up, around, and down the back, or up and down the back and front of the legs. The faster the strokes the more stimulating the massage will be; the slower the more relaxing. Put more effort into the upward stroke.

Petrissage

The muscles are squeezed or rolled, rather like kneading bread. This stroke is used on the legs, buttocks, back, and upper chest. If you are using this technique on the legs, place your hands on either side of the leg and dig in deep with the heel of your palm, moving your hands slowly out in opposite directions.

Tapotement

Also known as hacking or chopping, this involves lightly beating the body with the sides of your hands. Keep your fingers, hands and wrists relaxed and don't raise them more than 4 in (10 cm) above the body. This technique should be used on the fleshy parts, such as the buttocks and thighs.

Frottage

Sometimes called friction, frottage is used to release specific areas of tension, usually on the back and shoulders, where tightness accumulates. Using your thumb and index finger, press down on a point that feels knotted and tense, then rotate the pad for around 10 seconds. Repeat this three or four times, finishing with gentle stroking movements.

Cupping

Cup your hands with your fingers and thumbs tightly closed, as if you were cupping them to catch water, and strike the body with your hollowed palms. This works well for fleshy parts of the body.

Massage techniques

A sensitive and skillful massage is enjoyable both physically and emotionally. With each stroke you can feel the muscles relax and any anxiety and tension drain away. As such, it is wonderful for stress-related conditions such as headaches and insomnia, backaches, strains, sciatica, stress-related asthma and eczema, irritable bowel syndrome, constipation, and digestive upsets.

To give or receive a massage you will need a firm surface, such as a table or the floor, to work on. (A table is best because it is easier for the person giving the massage to move around it.) You will also need oil, cream, or talcum powder to lubricate your hands and a large towel. Choose a quiet warm room—the more rested and at peace you and your partner feel the better.

The following massage techniques are for two people and the person being massaged should be lying down. Pour about a teaspoon of vegetable oil into the palm of one hand and rub your hands together to warm the oil before you begin applying any strokes.

Chest massage

A chest massage may help ease asthma symptoms. Begin by loosening the back muscles by slow gliding effleurage strokes, then knead around the shoulders, and use cupping strokes over the middle back area. Use friction techniques in the

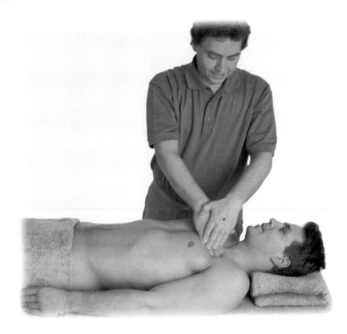

When giving a massage, you should try to maintain a fairly upright and relaxed posture as you move your hands up the chest.

upper chest, just below the neck bone, finishing with light kneading or fanning strokes over the upper chest.

Shoulder massage

To relax your partner's shoulders, use smooth fanning strokes from the collar bone, around the shoulders, and up the back of the neck to the base of the skull. Press down on the shoulders with your palms to open out the chest and improve breathing. Hold the shoulders down for about 10 seconds before releasing slowly.

Back massage

This is an all-purpose relaxing massage. Kneeling at your partner's head, place your hands on either side of the spine at the top, then move them down, sweep them around, and back to the neck. Use kneading strokes to break up areas of tension around the shoulders and neck and use friction techniques down either side of the spine. Finish with long effleurage strokes.

Quick neck and shoulder massage

This can be done sitting down, through clothes. Use gentle fanning strokes from the neck, over the shoulders, and down the back. After a few minutes, squeeze the band of muscle that runs from the neck to shoulder and work on any tight spots between the shoulders using your thumb pads. Place your hands on the shoulders, reach down with your thumbs, and gently but firmly roll the flesh upward.

WARNING

Seek medical advice before having a massage if you have a heart problem, bronchitis, weepy eczema, varicose veins, inflammation of the veins (phlebitis), acute back pain, blood clots (thrombosis), a fever, or if you are in the first three months of pregnancy. Don't massage any bruises or swellings or muscle tears that are severe and painful.

Healing

The "laying on of hands," or healing, exists in most cultures, and its roots lie in early religions, magic practices, and shamanism. Throughout history individuals with the power to heal have been (and still are) singled and out and revered.

You will usually sit in a chair for a healing session, though it can be done lying down.

The healer will either place his hands on you, using them as conduits to channel the healing energy into your body, or connect to the aura in the space around you.

Healing is the restoration to health of one individual by another through channeling healing energy. This is done either by the laying on of hands or from a distance. Healers believe that energy exists all around a person and that they can channel this energy to the patient to stimulate his or her own natural resources to restore well-being.

Visiting a healer

Most healers work from their home or are based at a healing center. The ambience will be relaxing, perhaps with incense or gentle music. The first session will last

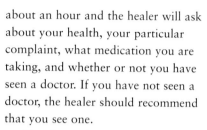

about an hour and the healer will ask about your health, your particular complaint, what medication you are taking, and whether or not you have seen a doctor. If you have not seen a doctor, the healer should recommend that you see one.

You do not have to concentrate—all the work is done by the healer. After spending a few moments mentally attuning himself to you, the healer will then place his hands on your body—sometimes on a diseased part, such as a patch of eczema—or pass them over you, a few inches away from your body.

The actual healing lasts around 15 minutes, though it can be shorter. The healer's hands may feel hot and you may feel a tingling sensation, freezing cold, or a feeling of deep relaxation.

Healers will say that their powers are a mystery—they are just conduits for an energy that comes from the cosmos and is emitted from the body. Many doctors say that healing is just placebo response at work, in other words, if you feel that some treatment will do you good, it probably will.

For such an esoteric therapy, there is a vast amount of research into healing. No reputable healer would claim to cure, but healers say there is no limit on the conditions that can benefit from healing. It is probably best used for chronic conditions, such as eczema, chronic fatigue syndrome, and mental conditions such as anxiety and depression.

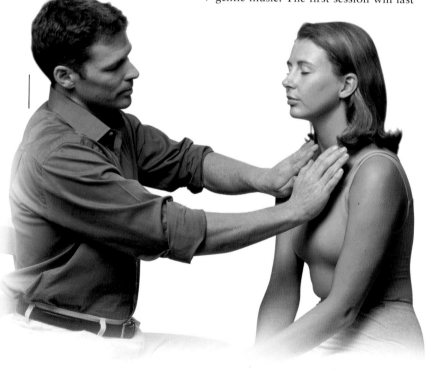

DIFFERENT TYPES OF HEALING

SPIRITUAL HEALING	A spiritual healer believes the healing energy comes from a divine source, usually, though not always, God, and healing takes place through the laying on of hands. It does not matter if the person who is receiving the healing has any faith.
PSYCHIC HEALING	This is a gift that only a few people achieve, usually when they have reached a high level of consciousness. Yogis and ascetics may achieve this after many years of meditation and contemplative thought; some people are just born with a gift and can harness the healing energy more effectively than others, with little or no conscious self-development.
FAITH HEALING	This usually takes place in a group and often in a religious context, such as during a church service. Unlike spiritual healing, it requires the person being healed to have a certain amount of faith in the powers of the person healing them. It is based on faith and trust in the power of the healer.
AURA HEALING	Healers claim to see bands of changing color radiating from the body, the aura, which reflect a person's health and mood. Kirlian photography, developed in the 1930s, clearly shows some kind of electronic, magnetic energy around the body, which can be recorded with photographic equipment. Aura healers believe that the colors emanate from the seven chakras, swirling vortices of energy that run down the body. Aura healers will place their hands on or near the person and visualize a healing color.
ABSENT HEALING	You can be healed at a distance, usually at a prearranged time, and the healer (either one person or a group of people) will visualize healing energy transferring from himself or themselves to you. Prayer falls into this category.
THERAPEUTIC TOUCH	This is a form of healing used by health care professionals. It is widely used in hospitals, particularly in the US, and is used in the treatment of patients who would find direct touch too painful. The healer works just above the surface of the body and the experience is believed to be deeply relaxing for the patient.
REIKI	Japanese Reiki is a form of touch therapy that involves the therapist treating a part of the body by laying their hands on or close to the part of the body that is painful. Practitioners claim that energy will start to flow through the hands into your body.

Reflexology

*R*eflex zone therapy, or reflexology, is a treatment in which the practitioner applies pressure to specific points, or reflexes, on the soles of the feet—and sometimes the hands and face—which are said to be related to various parts of the body.

You may be asked to sit or lie down for a reflexology massage. Some therapists massage only the feet; others work points on the hands and feet corresponding to the same zones, in succession.

A reflexology massage is intended to boost energy levels and restore emotional well-being, as well as alleviating specific conditions. Massaging the feet is practiced as part of Traditional Chinese Medicine and was also used by the early Egyptians and Native Americans. The art was rediscovered in 1913 by Dr. William Fitzgerald, an American ear, nose, and throat specialist, who found that applying pressure to particular parts of the hand and foot numbed the ear, allowing him to perform minor surgery without having to use anesthetics.

In 1917, he published *Zone Therapy*, in which he described his theory that the body could be divided into 10 equal and vertical zones and that pressure on one part of a zone could affect everything else in that zone. His ideas were popularized in the 1930s by American physiotherapist Eunice Ingham and one of her students, Doreen Bayley. Reflexology is now popular around the world and is frequently used in hospitals.

The theory

Reflexologists believe the body is divided into 10 reflex zones, or pathways, which run from the feet up the body to the head and down to the hands. There are reflexes on the soles of the foot, palms of the hands, ears, tongue, and head, which correspond to every part of the body, rather like a map. The right foot and hand represent the right side of the body, while the left hand and foot represent the left side of the body.

When a reflexologist works on particular points on the feet, he or she can stimulate organs in the same zone of the body into self-healing. As in acupuncture, in reflexology disease is seen as stemming from blocked energy pathways. Reflexology can be used to clear these pathways and restore the flow of energy. When there is an imbalance, crystalline deposits of calcium and uric acid build up at the nerve endings at the relevant reflex point, and practitioners can feel this.

Reflexology is good for stress-related conditions, particularly migraines, headaches, back problems, and digestive disorders such as irritable bowel

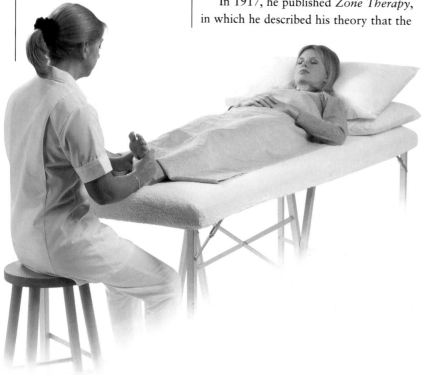

syndrome. Practitioners say that it can also help asthma and skin disorders, such as eczema and psoriasis.

There is good deal of anecdotal evidence that reflexology works, particularly in treating stress-related conditions, but there is no scientific evidence to back up its claims. However, various studies have shown that regular reflexology sessions can help constipation and premenstrual tension. It is also known that there are thousands of nerve endings on the soles of each foot and stimulating these may send messages to different parts of your body, stimulating the circulatory and lymphatic systems, which in turn will improve your health.

Visiting a reflexologist

At the first session, which will last about an hour, the practitioner will question you about your health and lifestyle and ask you to relax in a reclining chair or on a couch with your feet slightly raised and your shoes and socks or panty hose removed. The practitioner will wipe and dust your feet with talcum powder before beginning. Most therapists work on the feet, but they can also work on the hands and sometimes the face.

Reflexologists say they can feel a slight swelling, which indicates a weakness in a particular part of the body. These swellings are crystalline deposits, and gentle pressure breaks them down and sets the healing process in motion.

If you have eczema the reflexologist may massage areas relating to the digestive system, such as the liver and kidneys, and the adrenal and pituitary glands. For asthma, the therapist may apply pressure to the reflex point relating to the solar plexus, encouraging the diaphragm and the lungs to relax.

After massaging the feet, the practitioner works up each zone in the foot stimulating the reflexes. He or she will use a variety of techniques of which caterpillarlike movements are the most common. This technique involves the reflexologist pressing the thumb or index finger into your foot, easing the pressure, moving the finger or thumb forward a little, and then pressing again.

If there is an energy blockage, your foot may feel tender, even rather painful, and the reflexologist will use gentle pressure to remove the blockage. The practitioner will intersperse compression with gentle massage. Reflexology treats you on a number of levels simultaneously and influences emotional and spiritual disorders as well as physical problems.

Most people feel relaxed after a reflexology session, but you may have a cough, rash, headache, or want to urinate more frequently. Reflexologists say that these are signs that toxins are being eliminated from the body. Your symptoms may become slightly worse for a short time after a session.

The number of relexology sessions you have depends on your overall health, but several may be needed before you feel a change. You do not have to be ill to visit a reflexologist; those in good health can relax and enjoy the massage.

Find out more

Acupressure 108
Chinese herbal medicine 112

VACUFLEX

This is a high-tech form of reflexology in which the feet are stimulated by vacuum pressure. It employs a pair of felt boots from which the air has been sucked by a pump, and the whole foot is treated in just five minutes. When the boots are removed, any red marks left on the feet indicate spots that need further treatment with special suction pads.

Biofeedback

The theory that individuals can become aware of, and exert some control over, involuntary bodily functions, such as heart rate, blood pressure, and muscle tension is at the heart of the technique of biofeedback.

Biofeedback is not a therapy in itself, but a means of monitoring your bodily functions through the use of other therapies such as meditation, autogenic training, and relaxation techniques. To learn to modify involuntary bodily functions, you need first to be given and then to monitor signals relating to the part of your body you are trying to control. These "feedback" signals, such as electronic responses from your muscles, are recorded on a biofeedback machine.

Although the technique dates back to the 1930s, the term "biofeedback" was coined in 1969. It was initially used to describe laboratory procedures that trained research subjects to alter their brain activity, muscle tension, heart rate, movement in the gut, stomach acidity, and other bodily functions that are normally controlled by the body's autonomic nervous system.

By hooking yourself up to a biofeedback device and altering subtle bodily functions, you can reduce your muscle tension, thereby alleviating all stress-related conditions, such as headaches, migraines, anxiety, insomnia, high blood pressure, irritable bowel syndrome, and asthma and allergies.

Visiting a practitioner

A biofeedback practitioner will show you how to use the machine, of which there are several types, and you will be wired up so that your bodily functions can be measured. An electroencephalograph (EEG) records your brain waves; an electromyograph (EMG) measures your muscle activity; and an electrocardiograph (ECG) monitors your heart rate. Heat changes in the skin are measured with a heat-temperature gauge and the skin's electrical conductivity is tested with an electrical skin response sensor (ESR).

Once the monitors are in place, you will be taught simple relaxation and breathing techniques so that you can control your body's responses. When you are relaxed you will see an increase in the number of alpha brain waves, a slowing down of the heart rate, and a decrease in sweat gland activity.

Biofeedback trains you to modify these bodily functions without the use of the biofeedback device and it takes about six sessions before you have fully grasped the technique. This is not as easy as it sounds. Many people find it hard to alter their involuntary functions without a machine to tell them how they are doing.

There is a huge body of scientific evidence—some 2,500 research papers in all—that supports the efficacy of biofeedback for various conditions. One study on the effect of biofeedback on asthma patients monitored 22 children who used deep muscle relaxation prompted by biofeedback responses. The asthmatic children were compared with a similar group who had no therapy. The children who were using biofeedback techniques showed improvements in peak flow rates and a reduction in the use of steroid medication and the number of admissions into a hospital.

Hypnotherapy

In the trancelike hypnotic state of mind you become highly receptive to suggestion. Once you are in this state, the therapist will make suggestions to help you control your symptoms or change your responses to them.

Hypnosis is a natural state. Most people daydream—fall into a self-hypnotic trancelike state—several times a day. A child's daydream can be so vivid that it can take the place of reality. Nine out of 10 people can be hypnotized by a skilled hypnotherapist. However, those who need to be in control are difficult to hypnotize.

No one really knows how hypnotism works. While you may feel drowsy during hypnotherapy, hypnosis is not a form of sleep. Some doctors believe it is an intense form of relaxation; others that it is an altered state of consciousness, where the brain shuts off nerves supplying sensory information. Another theory is that it activates the creative right side of the brain, while shutting down the left side which deals with logical analytical thought.

Relaxation is at the heart of hypnotherapy, consequently it is of most use in treating stress-related conditions such as hypertension, migraines, tension headaches, and irritable bowel syndrome. It is a powerful and effective treatment for asthma and allergies. It can affect skin temperature, as well as the sensitive bronchi and gut, and it can reduce the symptoms of skin allergens.

Regular use of hypnosis can help you if you have asthma. You can stop an attack at its start with self-hypnosis, and hypnotherapy can alleviate the stress associated with an attack. Hypnotherapy has reduced hospital admission rates, length of stay, and steroid use. Most people with asthma who undergo hypnotherapy feel that their symptoms have improved.

Visiting a hypnotherapist

After taking a medical history, the therapist may suggest you are feeling tired and heavy, and will probably use an image—a flight of steps or a walk into a forest—to "count" you into a deeper trance. When you reach the center of the forest or bottom of the staircase, you will feel detached from the real world.

When you are in a deep trance, the therapist will make suggestions or ask you to imagine a scenario. If you have eczema, you may be asked to imagine bathing in a cool stream. If you are stressed, you may visualize opening the gates to a dam. Some hypnotherapists plant a suggestion that your symptoms will fade and this is usually combined with general suggestions of well-being and self-confidence. To return to consciousness—which you can do at any time—the hypnotherapist will guide you up the stairs or back through the forest.

A course usually comprises six hour-long sessions, during which you will be taught how to relax and hypnotize yourself.

WARNING

It is wise to be treated by a clinically trained hypnotherapist, in other words, a doctor, nurse, or psychologist who has also been trained in hypnotherapy. Hypnotism is easy to learn, but the art—and therapeutic benefits—of hypnotherapy lies in knowing how to treat someone once they have been hypnotized.

Hypnosis may cause an abreaction, where old memories rise to the surface, causing distress. Be wary of hypnotherapists who want to recover "repressed" memories. Repressed memories, if they exist at all, are best recovered by an experienced psychotherapist.

Psychotherapy and counseling

The overall benefits to health due to psychotherapy and counseling may not seem as obvious as those derived from other therapies. However, there is little doubt that your emotional life affects how you feel physically as well as mentally.

It can be difficult to make the decision to see a counselor, but talking through your problems with someone who is uninvolved with them, and who is in no way judgmental, can be enormously helpful.

Many studies have shown that a positive outlook can help patients recover from illness, while those people who suppress their emotions, or who have no outlet for their feelings, make a poor recovery. Loss of hope, the traumatic loss of an important relationship through divorce or death, and being laid off at work often result in despair, which can lead to illness.

This is not to say that a happy positive disposition will necessarily cure your asthma or allergies, but the mind and body are linked and you can stimulate your own self-healing process. There is evidence that stress and your mood can have an impact on your airways and some scientists have identified people who are at particular risk from asthma. Denial, repressed hostility, and emotional immaturity have been associated with people who have poor control over their asthma.

There are hundreds of counseling techniques to treat psychological suffering or physical conditions that may have psychological roots. These therapies encourage you to talk openly about your innermost thoughts, fears, anxieties, and problems to a trained and experienced listener, who will guide you and help you find solutions to whatever is worrying you. You can be counseled on your own, with a partner, or in groups.

Psychotherapy is the treatment of emotional problems by psychological means. A trained person establishes a relationship with a client with the object of altering ways of behavior so that you can lead a more positive life.

Psychotherapy is a "talking" technique which is non-judgemental and respects the client's values. The relationship you develop with the therapist is probably more important than the theory that underpins it, but both require commitment and energy—a course of psychotherapy can be hard work.

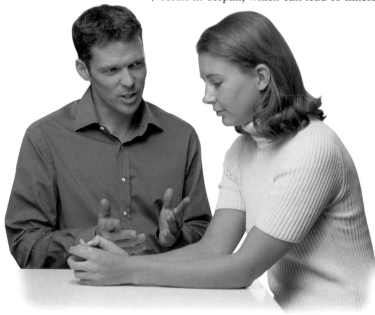

PSYCHIATRY AND PSYCHOTHERAPY

Psychotherapy is not the same as psychiatry. Psychotherapy is the study of human behavior, and treatment takes the form of getting you to understand your psychological problems by talking them through with a trained listener. Psychiatry is a medical discipline focusing on mental disorder, and treatment usually involves drug therapy. Psychiatrists are trained doctors.

TYPES OF THERAPY

PSYCHOANALYSIS	Psychoanalysts believe that the roots of unhappiness and anxieties lie in the subconscious. Sometimes they are buried so deeply that you forget them. However, these repressed emotions surface later in life as depression, anxiety, or stress-related illnesses, such as irritable bowel syndrome or migraines. Psychoanalysis attempts to unlock the key to your subconscious and repressed thoughts. Treatment may involve saying whatever comes into your mind. Freud set great store by this free association and he believed that this gave him clues to the subconscious mind. Your analyst may also analyze your dreams, since these may reveal hidden conflicts.
PSYCHODYNAMIC THERAPY	This approach stresses the importance of past experiences on your current behavior. The therapist will encourage you to talk about your childhood and your relationship with your parents and other people who were important in the past, as well as your work and family life. He will try to discover whether you are transferring feelings you had about people in your past to your current relationships. This should lead to a greater self-awareness and a resolution to current problems. Psychodynamic therapists often take a more active part in the sessions than psychoanalysts.
BEHAVIORAL THERAPY	The theory behind behavioral therapy is that all behavior is learned and so can be unlearned and new behavior acquired—without delving into the past. Behavioral therapy works on the basis that exposure to whatever you fear in a safe, controlled environment will render it less threatening and that desirable behavior can be rewarded. This form of therapy is particularly successful in treating anxiety, depression, obsessive behaviors, and phobias. For instance, if you have a phobia about spiders, your therapist might show you a picture of a spider first, then a film about spiders, and finally you will handle small and then large spiders.
COGNITIVE-BEHAVIORAL THERAPY	This type of therapy, sometimes simply called cognitive therapy, is based on the belief that the way you perceive the world influences your emotions and consequently your behavior. Someone suffering from depression may be locked in a spiral of negative thinking and believe that all undesirable events are his or her fault, while good experiences are pure chance. Through cognitive-behavioral therapy you will learn to challenge negative thought patterns and be taught how to think positively.
NEUROLINGUISTIC PROGRAMING (NLP)	NLP combines cognitive-behavioral techniques with hypnotherapy and other forms of psychotherapy and works on the principle that life experiences shape the way you see the world. A therapist will analyze how and why you have learned to behave as you do and you will be taught to change your behavior.
COUNSELING	Counseling has become enormously popular and many clinics and doctors' offices have a resident counselor. Counseling is usually most successful when it is applied to a specific problem, such as redundancy, relationship problems, or bereavement. Many stress-related conditions—and your allergies may be exacerbated by stress—clear up after discussing your problems and symptoms with a sympathetic and trained listener.

Choosing a practitioner

T*rying to find a complementary practitioner is not as easy as choosing a doctor. When you visit a doctor you can be certain that he or she is fully qualified, or else he or she would not be practicing. If you have any doubts you can check into a doctor's credentials and if you feel you have not been treated properly you can complain through established channels.*

In most of Europe, complementary practitioners must be registered, and only registered health professionals are allowed to practice. However, in the U.S. regulation varies, with each state legislating independently and on its own behalf. There is no nationwide body which oversees the registration of complementary therapists.

Personal recommendation is one of the best ways of finding a good complementary therapist, but you should still check his or her credentials. This is particularly important if you have decided to try a therapy that involves physical manipulation, such as chiropractic or osteopathy, or one that involves invasive techniques, such as herbal medicine where you swallow remedies, or acupuncture, where you are needled.

If your friends or colleagues are unable to help you, ask your doctor if he or she is able to recommend anyone. Or contact your local natural health center or health retail outlet. Sometimes places such as libraries have noticeboards on which people can advertise. Try chatting to the store assistants or librarians, since they may have had positive feedback about a particular practitioner. Most therapies will have a governing body that will monitor standards in that therapy and ensure that

Telephone the trade association of a particular therapy and ask them to send you a list of practitioners in your area. If possible, speak to your chosen therapist on the phone before booking a session.

the public is protected from unscrupulous therapists. It will publish a register of qualified practitioners—ask to consult this so that you can choose one who works in your area.

Such an organization will have fixed training standards, a code of practice and ethics, a complaints system, a disciplinary procedure, and effective sanctions, such as striking off a fraudulent practitioner, and a requirement for professional indemnity insurance. The organization in turn will most likely belong to an umbrella body, which holds details of different complementary therapy groups.

Choose a therapy you feel happy with. Don't try any therapy you are scared of. If you don't like needles, then acupuncture may not be right for you, though acupressure may suit you. If you are worried about drinking a concoction of strange herbs, then reflexology may be better for you than Western or Chinese herbal·medicine.

Checking practitioner's credentials

Before you book a treatment session with a therapist, have a chat with him or her on the phone or, better still, arrange to meet in person. You will be investing time and money in the treatment and putting your trust in this person so it is perfectly understandable for you to want to be happy with the arrangement.

A reputable practitioner will welcome your questions about credentials and, in

WARNING

Avoid practitioners who:
- *Make excessive claims about their therapy or who promise to cure you. No health practitioner—complementary or conventional—can guarantee a cure.*
- *Criticizes the work of other therapists.*
- *Tries to persuade you to stop seeing your doctor or stop taking your medication. Reputable practitioners work quite happily alongside conventional health professionals and many do so in hospitals and clinics.*
- *Is more expensive than other therapists and says you need a large number of treatment sessions before you will see any improvement.*

fact, you should be wary of any therapist unwilling to tell you precisely what their qualifications are. Even if the therapist tells you what his or her qualifications are, it might mean little to you, so check with that therapy's main professional body. You may find this listed in the telephone book, or ask at the library.

Questions to ask

Before you start on a course of complementary therapy, you should ask the practitioner the following:
- What are your qualifications and how long was your training?
- Are you registered with a reputable organization and what is its name?
- How long have you been practicing?
- What will the treatment involve?
- Is it the right therapy for my condition?
- How many sessions will I need?
- How much will it cost?
- Are you covered by professional indemnity insurance?

Relationship with practitioner

You may be having treatment over months, or even years, so it is important to feel comfortable with the practitioner and to trust him or her. For some

therapies, such as osteopathy or massage, close physical contact is involved, so you may want to be treated by someone of the same sex. If you feel uncomfortable when you meet the therapist there is little point in starting treatment. Do not feel shy or embarassed to say that you feel the treatment is not for you.

After your first session, ask yourself the following questions:
- Did I feel comfortable and relaxed with the practitioner?
- Did I have confidence in his or her ability and integrity?
- Did he or she answer my questions fully and to my satisfaction?
- Was I treated with respect?
- Was I given any literature either on the therapy or the practitioner to look through?

In the end, your choice of complementary therapist comes down to personal choice and circumstance. You may just not feel comfortable with a particular therapist, in spite of his or her speciality. In this case look for another.

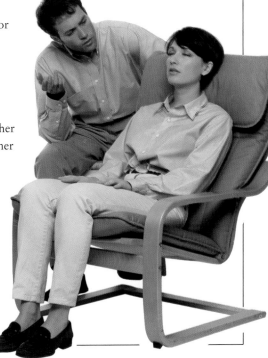

It is important that you trust a therapist totally and feel relaxed in his or her company

New directions

A growing body of evidence points to the fact that one of the underlying causes of asthma and allergies may be that children are too protected from infection and are not developing an immune system robust enough to fight off simple allergies.

The University of Southampton in the UK, one of the world's leading research centers into asthma and allergies, is working on a vaccine that could protect you from asthma and hay fever. Developed from a type of microbacteria, Mycobacterium vaccae, found naturally in the soil, the vaccine corrects imbalances in the immune system by stimulating your Th-1 cells (below) and reducing the number of Th-2 cells.

Recent research involving almost 2,000 patients showed that children who were given broad-spectrum antibiotics—for colds and chest complaints—are three times more likely to develop asthma, eczema and hay fever later in life.

The key to the allergic response is two types of cells produced by the immune system: Th-1 and Th-2. Th-1 cells are released when the body is invaded by bacteria and viruses; Th-2 cells tackle parasites. Both normally coexist in harmony. Scientists now believe that bacteria living in the gut help the immune system respond normally. If they are artificially removed, for instance by too many antibiotics, then a young child will end up producing too many Th-2 cells.

In other words, he or she will develop allergic reactions to many substances and may also develop asthma.

Hard evidence that chest infections protect against asthma comes from a study that has linked the decline of tuberculosis (TB) to a rise of the immune response to house dust mites, pollen, and other allergens. The study found that Japanese children with a strong immune response to TB were relatively insensitive to allergens such as dust mites and pollen and less prone to asthma. Immunization with harmless bacteria related to TB may thus help in treating allergies.

Doctors also believe that babies in the West have too "sterile" a diet and that the immune system is being given little to do. Instead of being bombarded with bacteria, it remains unchallenged and so becomes alerted by things that are not harmful, like pollen.

Many of these new theories hold the key to future drugs and vaccines, but until they are developed, it is worth remembering that when it comes to colds, sore throats, and mild chest infections, it may be best to let nature take its course, to allow your child to build up immunities.

Asthma

Two new asthma drugs have been launched recently, which could make a difference to many asthma sufferers. Zarfirlukast (Accolate) and montelukast sodium (Singulair) belong to a new class of anti-inflammatory medication, the first new type of drug to be launched in 20

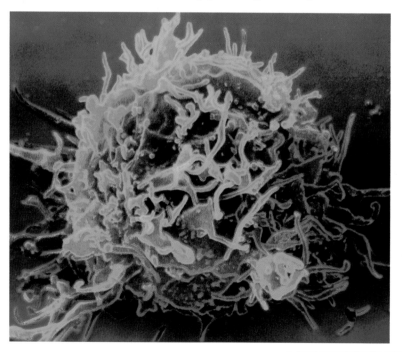

ANTIALLERGY VACCINE

Scientists are developing a vaccine that could prevent allergies such as hay fever, allergic asthma, and severe reactions to food, drugs, animals, and insect stings. The vaccine is being developed by a British biopharmaceutical company in conjunction with the pharmaceutical giant SmithKline Beecham, one of the world's largest manufacturer of vaccines.

The vaccine works by blocking the body's immune response to allergens and preventing the release of histamine, which causes the allergy symptoms. Because the vaccine stops this spurt of chemicals, it works for all allergies—from childhood asthma and hay fever to severe food allergies and reactions to insect stings that could result in anaphylactic shock.

Two clinical trials have been carried out at an internationally recognized allergy center in Poland. The first involved 20 hay-fever sufferers. It worked and there were no reported side effects. The second was carried out on 13 people with histories of severe food allergies, two of whom had suffered from anaphylactic shock. The patients were vaccinated and then given the foods that triggered their allergy.

years. Both work by targeting natural body chemicals called leukotrienes, which are released by the body's immune system in response to allergens, such as house dust mites, and set off an asthma attack.

The leukotrienes play an important role in inflaming and narrowing the airways during an attack and are believed to be nearly 10,000 times more potent a bronchoconstrictor than histamine. They also have been linked to a number of inflammatory conditions.

Montelukast, taken as a pill once a day at bedtime, is a preventer and is suitable for adults and children as young as six with chronic mild to moderate asthma as an "add-on" medication, in other words, in addition to your usual inhaled drug. It works by blocking the activity of leukotrienes.

Scientific trials show that it improves lung function, both daytime and night-time symptoms, and significantly reduces the symptoms of asthma brought on by exercise or aspirin. Researchers found that when a 10 mg dose was taken once a day 48 percent of those sufferers being tested had fewer asthma attacks than when they were just taking steroids alone.

Zarfirlukast also blocks the activity of leukotrienes. It is taken as a pill twice a day and is suitable for adults and children over 12. It targets leukotriene D4, to which people who have asthma are particularly sensitive and which contributes to mucus secretion, inflammation, and bronchoconstriction. Both drugs work differently from steroids and your usual reliever medication and if taken regularly reduce the need for bronchodilators and improve symptoms.

Doctors have also found when the long-acting bronchodilator eformoterol is combined with the inhaled steroid budesonide in a turbohaler, it can cut the number of asthma attacks by a third, compared with the same dose of the steroid alone.

Emergency treatment

What to do during an asthma attack

An asthma attack is serious. People do die from them, particularly older people. Asthma attacks can be mild, moderate, or severe and managing a severe attack is a job for a doctor. A severe attack should always be treated in a hospital; most people who die from asthma do so outside a hospital. It is vital to recognize the danger signs and to know how to react, when to call for help, and what to do until help arrives.

Early warning signs

Warning signs vary from person to person and you should never ignore them, particularly if you have a history of acute attacks. It is important to remember that sometimes you can have an attack with little or no warning.

The most common signs that herald an attack are:

- A tickly cough
- A strange or itchy sensation in the skin or nose
- Nausea or vomiting
- Light-headedness
- A worsening of your usual symptoms
- Disturbed sleep
- A need for more reliever medication

It can be difficult not to panic during an asthma attack, but you will help yourself by remaining calm. Sit upright with your head slightly forward, loosen clothing around your neck, and try to take deep breaths.

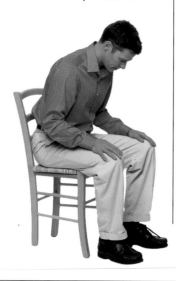

Call for a doctor when:

- The peak flow rate falls below 50 percent of your personal best.
- The symptoms are so severe that it is impossible to talk or finish a sentence.
- You have to sit or lie down.
- There is a bluish discoloration of the tongue or mouth, a sure sign that not enough oxygen is being taken in.
- You begin to sweat.
- You have a racing pulse (more than **120 beats** a minute for an adult and **140 beats** for a child).
- You are exhausted.
- Your usual medication gives no relief in the time frame stated on the package

What to do during an acute attack

- Take **15–30 puffs** of reliever medication.
  This is a high dose, but this is an emergency.
- Try to remain calm. This is easy to say and difficult to do, but overbreathing brought on by panic can make things worse.
- Sit upright, leaning slightly forward, and place your hands on your knees to support your chest. Don't lie down.
- Take slow, deep breaths.
- Loosen clothing around your neck.
- Try to drink warm water—rapid breathing will make your mouth dry.

If someone else is having an attack

- Try to remain calm and, if they can talk, listen to what they are saying. Ask them if they have any reliever inhaler and if they have help them to take large doses. If they have difficulty doing this, you can make an emergency spacer by rolling up a sheet of paper into a cone, placing it over their face and firing the inhaler every 10 seconds for 15–30 puffs.
- Don't put your arm around a child's shoulder because this can restrict breathing further.

Find out more

Extreme allergic reactions   30
Managing your asthma   74
Breathing techniques   86

Anaphylactic shock

Anaphylaxis is a life-threatening allergic reaction to a particular substance, often insect stings or certain foods, such as nuts. The only emergency treatment is epinephrine, usually administered by an epinephrine injection pen (EpiPen, Anapen, Min-i-jet), which works directly on the heart and lungs, thereby reversing the fatal effects of anaphylaxis.

If you have anaphylaxis, you should always carry your epinephrine pen with you—many people carry two. You should carry antihistamine tablets and wear a MedicAlert bracelet. Tell your friends and colleagues that you have anaphylaxis and show them how to use the autoinjector. If your child has anaphylaxis make sure teachers and friends know that he or she is at risk. Make sure that your child's teacher has an epinephrine pen for him or her.

Symptoms usually erupt within seconds of exposure to the allergen and include:

- Itching or a metallic taste in the mouth
- Swelling of the throat and mouth
- Difficulty in swallowing and breathing
- Flushing of the skin
- Abdominal cramps and nausea
- Hives anywhere on the body

How to use an epinephrine pen

If your partner, child, or a close friend has anaphylaxis you must know how to use the epinephrine pen.

- Take off the black top to expose the needle tip
- Press hard against the outer thigh, through clothing if necessary. This should activate the spring mechanism and inject the epinephrine
- Keep it against the thigh for at least 10 seconds
- Remove, and massage the area
- One dose is usually enough, but if symptoms don't get better after 10–15 minutes use a second pen
- **Call an ambulance immediately**

Glossary

Acupoint: a point along one of the body's meridians, which can be manipulated either by needles or by pressure to bring about health and well-being.

Adrenaline: the "fight or flight" hormone released by the adrenal glands in response to stress or fear.

Allergen: the tiny substances or particles you react to.

Alveoli: microscopic air sacs at the end of the bronchioles where oxygen is transferred to the bloodstream and carbon dioxide removed and passed out.

Anaphylaxis: a severe life-threatening allergic reaction.

Angioedema: a swelling of the tissues, particularly on the face, as a result of an allergic reaction.

Antibodies: cells produced by the immune system in response to a foreign substance.

Antihistamines: drugs that block the action of histamine and so alleviate the allergic symptoms.

Atopy/atopic: a family tendency to allergies; you may develop allergic conditions such as asthma, eczema, and hay fever.

Aura: an energy field that the body is believed to emit and that can be manipulated to bring about healing.

Autonomic nervous system: part of the nervous system responsible for involuntary muscle movement and the functioning of structures, such as the gut, eyes, the airway and blood vessels.

Beta-2 agonists: bronchodilating drugs that bind to special places or "receptors" in the bronchi, which makes them relax.

Bronchi/bronchioles: small thin-walled branches in the lungs that become inflamed during an asthma attack.

Celiac disease: a disease of the small intestine caused by intolerance to gluten.

Chakra: the body has seven chakras—spinning "wheels" of energy—along the spinal column through which life energy (prana), interacts with the body and mind.

Corticosteroids: chemicals produced naturally in the body by the adrenal glands and which are synthesized to produce anti-inflammatory drugs to alleviate allergic symptoms, particularly asthma, eczema, and hay fever.

Cyanosis: the bluish discoloration of the mouth and tongue during an acute asthma attack.

Dander: microscopic particles of animal fur, skin, and saliva that can trigger allergies.

Epinephrine: adrenaline.

FEV1 (forced expiratory volume in one second): the volume of air that you can force out of your lungs in one second after you've taken in a deep breath.

Gluten: a protein found in wheat, oats, barley, and rye.

Histamine: an inflammatory chemical released by the body during an allergic reaction. It stimulates mucus production and other allergic symptoms.

IgE (immunoglobulin E): the allergy antibody produced in large amounts by those with allergies.

Immune system: the body's defense against foreign substances, such as allergens, bacteria, and viruses.

Mast cells: cells activated by the allergy antibody IgE and containing granules, which cause the changes in the air passages characteristic of an asthma attack.

Meridians: in Chinese medicine, a network of invisible pathways, along which flows a life-energy or qi. When these are unbalanced, blocked, or stagnant you get sick.

Peak flow rate: a measurement of the strength of exhalation, used to judge the health of the lungs.

Pollen count: the number of pollen grains in a cubic meter of air. Below 50 is low; 200 and above is high.

Preventers: drugs, usually corticosteroids, which prevent the symptoms of asthma and reduce inflammation.

RAST (radioallergosorbant test): a blood test measuring the amount of IgE in the bloodstream when you are exposed to a particular allergen, such as pollen.

Relievers: drugs giving quick relief from asthma symptoms.

Rhinitis: inflammation of the nose, often caused by grass pollen.

Sinusitis: inflammation of the sinuses, hollow cavities linked to the nose and throat that, when inflamed, fill with mucus.

Smooth muscle: muscle in the air passages, blood-vessel walls, gut, and bladder that moves involuntarily.

Sympathetic nervous system: part of the autonomic nervous system, which prepares the body for "fight or flight" and dilates the bronchial passages.

T cells: cells put out by the immune system to fight foreign invaders, such as bacteria.

Urticaria: also called hives or nettle rash; swelling of the skin as a result of an allergic reaction.

Yin/yang: in Chinese medicine, a balance of energy. Yang is characterized by heat, movement, light, and energy; yin by darkness, inactivity, sluggishness, and deficiency.

Helpful organizations

ORGANIZATIONS IN THE U.S.A.

American Lung Association
432 Park Avenue South, 8th Floor
New York, New York 10016
800-LUNG-USA; 212-889-3370
www.lungusa.org

Asthma and Allergy Foundation of
America
1125 15th Street NW, Suite 502
Washington, DC 20005
800-7ASTHMA; 202-466-7643
www.aafa.org

Allergy and Asthma
Network/Mothers of Asthmatics,
Inc.
3554 Chain Bridge Road, Suite 200
Fairfax, VA 22030
800-878-4403; 703-385-4403
www.aanma.org

National Eczema Association for
Science and Education
1220 Southwest Morrison, Suite 443
Portland, OR 97205
800-818-7546;503-228-4430
www.eczema-assn.org

National Psoriasis Foundation
6600 SW 92nd Avenue, Suite 300
Portland, OR 97223
800-723-9166; 503-297-1545
www.psoriasis.org/npf.shtml

American Academy of Allergy,
Asthma and Immunology
611 E. Wells Street
Milwaukee, WI 53202
800-822-2762
www.aaaai.org

ORGANIZATIONS IN CANADA

Acupuncture Foundation of Canada
2131 Lawrence Avenue E, Suite 204
Scarborough, ON M1R 5G4
Tel: (416) 752-3988

Canadian Chiropractic Association
1396 Eglinton Avenue W
Toronto, ON M6C 2E4
Tel: (416) 781-5656

Reflexology Association of Canada
Box 110, 451 Turnberry Street
Brussels, ON N0G 1M0
Tel: (519) 887-9991

Canadian Association of
Homeopathic Physicians
10240A 152nd Street
Surrey, BC V3R 6N7
Tel: (604) 951-9987

Canadian Osteopathic Association
575 Waterloo Street
London, ON N6B 2R2
Tel: (519) 439-5521

The Canadian Association of Herbal
Practitioners
#400 - 1228 Kensington Road NW
Calgary, AB T2N 4P9
Tel: (403) 270-0936

Index